Social Perspectives on Trans Health

Transgender people are waiting to be seen in health care and waiting to be recognised as the legitimate experts on their own lives and needs. This book foregrounds empirically novel and conceptually groundbreaking sociological analyses of trans health care and experiences.

It draws together sociological contributions focused on the lives and perspectives of trans people to provide a vision of more equitable and affirming health and social care. Chapters explore how gender affirmation is imagined and enacted, and how trans people creatively and collectively work to secure the care they require in countries such as Australia, Aotearoa New Zealand, and the United Kingdom. Concluding with a commentary on trans health in the Global South by Professor Emerita Raewyn Connell, this book demonstrates the urgent need for radical sociopolitical transformation, grounded in a recognition of trans people as authorities in and on their own lives.

Social and health science students and researchers will be inspired by the critical perspectives this book provides on normative framings of gender and health, and health practitioners, policymakers and advocates will benefit from better understanding the challenges trans people face in securing safe and quality health care today. This book was originally published as a special issue of *Health Sociology Review.*

Christy E. Newman (they/them) is a social researcher of health, gender, and sexuality at the Centre for Social Research in Health, UNSW Sydney. As a queer/bi+ and non-binary person, they draw on both lived experience and research expertise in contributing to public discussions on diverse genders, sexualities, relationships, and families.

Anthony K J Smith (he/him) is a sociologist of health specialising in HIV and LGBTQ+ communities. He is employed as a postdoctoral researcher at the Centre for Social Research in Health, UNSW Sydney. Anthony is Editorial Advisory Board member of *Health Sociology Review* and Associate Editor of *Sexual Health.*

Elizabeth Duck-Chong (she/they) is a writer, researcher, and filmmaker who works across LGBTQ+ sexual health, advocacy, and education. In previous roles, Liz has set up peer-based services, and was the lead writer of transgender health and well-being platform TransHub. Liz is also Board Director of the Trans Justice Project.

Son Vivienne (they/them) is CEO of Transgender Victoria and has lived experience as a trans-masc non-binary, pansexual and neurodivergent parent, bee-keeper, and gardener. They have a background in media production and their most recent book is *Queering Safe Spaces: Being Brave Beyond Binaries*.

Cristyn Davies (she/her) is a research fellow in the Speciality of Child and Adolescent Health at the University of Sydney, Australia, and co-chair of the Research Committee of the Australian Professional Association for Trans Health. Cristyn has expertise in gender and sexuality diverse young people and culturally safe health care.

Kerry H. Robinson (she/they) is a sociologist in the School of Social Sciences at Western Sydney University, Australia. Kerry's research expertise includes LGBTQ+ health and well-being, gender and sexuality subjectivity in childhood, gender and sexuality-based violence, and sexuality education.

Peter Aggleton (he/him) has a background in the social sciences as applied to well-being, education, and health. He holds senior professorial positions at a number of universities including UCL in London, The Australian National University in Canberra, and UNSW Sydney.

Social Perspectives on Trans Health

Edited by
Christy E. Newman, Anthony K J Smith, Elizabeth Duck-Chong, Son Vivienne, Cristyn Davies, Kerry H. Robinson and Peter Aggleton

Routledge
Taylor & Francis Group
LONDON AND NEW YORK

First published 2024
by Routledge
4 Park Square, Milton Park, Abingdon, Oxon OX14 4RN

and by Routledge
605 Third Avenue, New York, NY 10158

Routledge is an imprint of the Taylor & Francis Group, an informa business

British Library Cataloguing in Publication Data
A catalogue record for this book is available from the British Library

ISBN13: 978-1-032-72242-9 (hbk)
ISBN13: 978-1-032-72243-6 (pbk)
ISBN13: 978-1-032-72244-3 (ebk)

DOI: 10.4324/9781032722443

Typeset in Minion Pro
by Newgen Publishing UK

Publisher's Note
The publisher accepts responsibility for any inconsistencies that may have arisen during the conversion of this book from journal articles to book chapters, namely the inclusion of journal terminology.

Contents

Citation Information

The chapters in this book were originally published in the journal *Health Sociology Review*, volume 30, issue 1 (2021). When citing this material, please use the original page numbering for each article, as follows:

Introduction

Waiting to be seen: social perspectives on trans health
Christy E. Newman, Anthony K J Smith, Elizabeth Duck-Chong, Son Vivienne, Cristyn Davies, Kerry H. Robinson and Peter Aggleton
Health Sociology Review, volume 30, issue 1 (2021), pp. 1–8

Chapter 1

Support for parents/carers of primary school aged gender diverse children in England, UK: a mixed-method analysis of experiences with health services
Bridgette Rickett, Katherine Johnson, Helen Ingle and Martel Reynolds
Health Sociology Review, volume 30, issue 1 (2021), pp. 9–24

Chapter 2

'A little bubble of utopia': constructions of a primary care-based pilot clinic providing gender affirming hormone therapy
Alex Ker, Gloria Fraser, Theresa Fleming, Cathy Stephenson, Anny da Silva Freitas, Richard Carroll, Thomas K. Hamilton and Antonia C. Lyons
Health Sociology Review, volume 30, issue 1 (2021), pp. 25–40

Chapter 3

Ontologies of transition(s) in healthcare practice: examining the lived experiences and representations of transgender adults transitioning in healthcare
Adam Shepherd and Benjamin Hanckel
Health Sociology Review, volume 30, issue 1 (2021), pp. 41–57

Chapter 4

Expanding and improving trans affirming care in Australia: experiences with healthcare professionals among transgender young people and their parents
Clare Bartholomaeus, Damien W. Riggs and Annie Pullen Sansfaçon
Health Sociology Review, volume 30, issue 1 (2021), pp. 58–71

Chapter 5

Not your unicorn: trans dating app users' negotiations of personal safety and sexual health
Kath Albury, Christopher Dietzel, Tinonee Pym, Son Vivienne and Teddy Cook
Health Sociology Review, volume 30, issue 1 (2021), pp. 72–86

Chapter 6

Transgender health: on a world scale
Raewyn Connell
Health Sociology Review, volume 30, issue 1 (2021), pp. 87–94

For any permission-related enquiries please visit:
www.tandfonline.com/page/help/permissions

Notes on Contributors

Peter Aggleton, Centre for Social Research in Health, UNSW Sydney, Sydney, Australia; School of Sociology, The Australian National University, Canberra, Australia.

Kath Albury, Media and Communication, Swinburne University of Technology, Hawthorn, Australia.

Clare Bartholomaeus, College of Education, Psychology and Social Work, Flinders University, Adelaide, Australia.

Richard Carroll, Centre for Endocrine, Diabetes, and Obesity Research, Wellington Regional Hospital, Wellington, New Zealand.

Raewyn Connell, Professor Emerita, University of Sydney and Life Member, National Tertiary Education Union, Sydney, Australia.

Teddy Cook, ACON, Sydney, Australia.

Anny da Silva Freitas, Mauri Ora Student Health and Counselling Services, Victoria University of Wellington, Wellington, New Zealand.

Cristyn Davies, Discipline of Child and Adolescent Health, Faculty of Medicine and Health, University of Sydney, Sydney, Australia.

Christopher Dietzel, Department of Integrated Education, McGill University, Montreal, Canada.

Elizabeth Duck-Chong, Independent Researcher, Sydney, Australia.

Theresa Fleming, School of Health, Victoria University of Wellington, Wellington, New Zealand.

Gloria Fraser, School of Psychology, Victoria University of Wellington, Wellington, New Zealand.

Thomas K. Hamilton, OutLine Aotearoa, Auckland, New Zealand.

Benjamin Hanckel, Institute for Culture and Society, Western Sydney University, Sydney, Australia.

Helen Ingle, North Yorkshire County Council, Leeds, UK.

Katherine Johnson, Global, Urban and Social Studies, RMIT University, Melbourne, Australia.

Alex Ker, School of Social and Cultural Studies, Victoria University of Wellington, Wellington, New Zealand.

Antonia C. Lyons, School of Health, Victoria University of Wellington, Wellington, New Zealand.

Christy E. Newman, Centre for Social Research in Health, UNSW Sydney, Sydney, Australia.

Annie Pullen Sansfaçon, School of Social Work, University of Montreal, Montreal, Canada.

Tinonee Pym, Media and Communication, Swinburne University of Technology, Hawthorn, Australia.

Martel Reynolds, Leeds Business School, Leeds Beckett University, Leeds, UK.

Bridgette Rickett, Psychology, Leeds Beckett University, Leeds, UK.

Damien W. Riggs, College of Education, Psychology and Social Work, Flinders University, Adelaide, Australia.

Kerry H. Robinson, School of Social Sciences, Western Sydney University, Sydney, Australia.

Adam Shepherd, King's College London, London, UK.

Anthony K J Smith, Centre for Social Research in Health, UNSW Sydney, Sydney, Australia.

Cathy Stephenson, Mauri Ora Student Health and Counselling Services, Victoria University of Wellington, Wellington, New Zealand.

Son Vivienne, Thorne Harbour Health, Melbourne, Australia and Transgender Victoria, Melbourne, Australia.

Introduction – Waiting to be seen: social perspectives on trans health

Christy E. Newman, Anthony K J Smith, Elizabeth Duck-Chong, Son Vivienne, Cristyn Davies, Kerry H. Robinson and Peter Aggleton

Sociologists have always had rich and sometimes controversial material to explore within the 'contentious epistemological space' (Brosnan & Kirby, 2016, p. 139) of health and medicine, but the field of trans[1] health has come to represent one of most highly contested of these domains today. When we first came together as a coalition of Australian cis and trans researchers to lead this special issue of *Health Sociology Review*, we were keenly aware of the tensions between those seeking to promote and to undermine a gender affirming approach to trans health. As we write this introduction, it seems almost an understatement to suggest that these conflicts are intensifying, with ever more distressing and harmful effects for trans people around the world.

A broad clinical consensus exists in support of the standard of care advanced by the World Professional Association for Transgender Health, first published in 1979, which requires all those involved in delivering health care to 'assist transsexual, transgender, and gender non-conforming people with safe and effective pathways to achieving lasting personal comfort with their gendered selves, in order to maximise their overall health, psychological well-being, and self-fulfilment' (WPATH, 2011, p. 1). For some trans people, hormone therapy and/or surgical procedures may be desired to align physical characteristics with gender identity (Cheung, Wynne, Erasmus, Murray, & Zajac, 2019), but trans advocates and researchers have worked hard to challenge the assumption that medical gender affirmation is desired by all. Health professionals are essential in providing appropriate forms of general health care to trans people in every context, and in supporting the process of social affirmation, which could include changes to names, pronouns, presentation, voice and relationships, and overcoming the many and complex hurdles to legal recognition and affirmation (ACON, 2020; Vincent, 2018).

But despite this robust and multidisciplinary consensus on best practice in trans health, a minority of critical voices seek to recast this field as holding the potential to do harm (for a recent summary, see: Pearce, Erikainen, & Vincent, 2020). This creates ongoing uncertainty for trans people regarding their right to access to the health care they need (Ashley, 2019; Pearce, 2018). As recent legal cases in both the United Kingdom (UK) and Australia have demonstrated, access to gender affirming care for minors, including puberty blockers and hormones, has become a site of extreme contention, creating immense and prolonged anxiety for those waiting to access these forms of care (AusPATH, 2020; WPATH, 2020). We know from repeated studies that trans people report some of the highest rates of mental health issues, including suicidal ideation, of any population, providing further evidence for the significance of attending to and securing their holistic health care needs (see, for example: Byron et al., 2017; Callander et al., 2019; Kang et al., 2018; Robinson, Bansel, Denson, Ovenden, & Davies, 2014; Strauss et al., 2017; Treharne, Riggs, Ellis, Flett, & Bartholomaeus, 2020).

Achieving health equity for trans people will require an ambitious combination of political will, community support and robust health systems. Even in Australia, where there is arguably a well-developed approach to providing gender affirming forms of health care, access depends on age, location, citizenship status, and financial capacity (particularly to gender affirming surgery which is not subsidised by the publicly funded health system), as well as the intensive labour of health care consumers in identifying and securing access to appropriate care providers (Davies, 2019; Newman, Prankumar et al., 2020). Too often, trans people report encounters with clinicians and allied health professionals who are unprepared for providing the care that is needed. For example, the phenomenon of 'trans broken arm syndrome' describes the experience of trans people being asked unnecessary questions about their gender when seeking care for something entirely unrelated (e.g. Newman, MacGibbon et al., 2020). Clinicians unfamiliar with trans health matters have also been critiqued for their 'inappropriate curiosity' (Shepherd, Hanckel, & Guise, 2019) when a trans person presents to them, requiring the service user to educate and reassure them, rather than the other way around, and perpetuating the circumstances in which potentially traumatising conversations and unnecessary examinations continue to be conducted (Sbragia & Vottero, 2020).

Perhaps unsurprisingly, then, many trans people describe being hyper conscious of what they should fear, and how they must perform, in seeking to access the health care they desire (e.g. Aizura, 2018; Ashley, 2019; Johnson, 2019; shuster, 2019). In too many cases, trans people avoid engaging with the care they need until their health has been significantly compromised (Vermeir, Jackson, & Marshall, 2018). While alternative networks of care and support within trans and queer communities fill the gaps in formal health and social support services at times of particular vulnerability and need (Hines, 2007), they are rarely resourced. As Hil Malatino (2020) describes: 'For many of us, surviving this process means committing to forms of healing that are unthinkable, indeed impossible, without care webs'. There is clearly an urgent need for increased resourcing in the field of trans health, and improved education embedded in both the initial training and ongoing professional development of all health and medical professionals (Blakey & Treharne, 2019; Davies et al., forthcoming; Stryker, Pallerla, & Pickle, 2020). But there is also a need for far greater recognition of the precarious social, legal and economic position of many trans people which impacts profoundly on health and wellbeing (Robinson et al., 2020; Winter et al., 2016).

As annually reported on Trans Day of Remembrance, the numbers of trans people known to have been murdered continues to increase each year, particularly women of colour and sex workers, and these numbers exclude the many people misgendered after death, or whose deaths are not reported in coronial data systems (TGEU, 2020). There are often substantial tensions between relevant national and local (eg. state, provincial, municipal) legal and policy frameworks, particularly with respect to identity documentation, which can expose trans people to increased surveillance and stigmatisation by law enforcement, administrative systems and social services (Wundram Pimentel & Leonardo Segura, 2018). As Raewyn Connell (2021) argues in the Invited Commentary included at the end of this special issue, many trans people live in conditions of chronic precarity, poverty, violence, and over-policing around the world; issues that can only be addressed through radical sociopolitical transformation, well beyond the question of what comprises best practice health care.

For this special issue, we aimed to build on the rapidly growing field of sociological research on trans lives and issues (e.g. Schilt & Lagos, 2017; Sumerau, 2020) by disseminating a call for papers examining the diverse and urgent range of health care and support issues experienced by trans and gender diverse people across the world. We made clear that we hoped to feature authorship groups which represented both established and emerging researchers in the trans health field, including trans collaborators and authors. As Scheim et al. (2019) have reminded those responsible for shaping professional cultures in the field of HIV research, the maxim 'nothing about us without us' valued in many other fields of social activism must always be prioritised in trans health also.

We are particularly grateful to the five authorship groups featured here for persevering through the review process during the COVID-19 crisis (Lupton, 2020). Perhaps compounded by the impacts, we received fewer submissions from non-English speaking settings than hoped, and the final five papers come from only Australia, Aotearoa New Zealand and the UK. We want to make clear, however, that trans health is an issue relevant to every country, society and context (e.g. Appenroth & Varela, forthcoming; Do & Nguyen, 2020). Nonetheless, despite their restricted geographic reach, the combination of these five papers address a diversity of topics, approaches and settings.

In reflecting on the observations made in these papers, we are struck by the repeated reference to the central metaphor of 'waiting to be seen', which captures a number of aspects of the way trans health is conceptualised and enacted today. The first is the most direct interpretation, recognising that in many parts of the world, too many trans people are quite literally *waiting to be seen by the care providers* they desire to access. In addition to the internal health system issues impacting care provision, accessing care requires capital of a variety of kinds: the social and mental health capital required to successfully navigate a series of complex professional and regulatory hurdles within an ever-shifting medicolegal landscape, the financial capital for negotiating travel costs and time away from work, and cultural capital in understanding how best to represent and communicate care needs, adapted to the conventions and preferences of different health care disciplines and environments (e.g. Aizura, 2018; Kang et al., 2018; Koch, McLachlan, Victor, Westcott, & Yager, 2020; Robinson et al., 2020).

These issues are explored in the contribution from Rickett et al (2020), who discuss the findings from a survey of the support needs of parents and carers of primary school aged gender diverse children living in Scotland, England and Wales. Following Plummer (1995), the authors argue that 'we are currently witnessing an important shift in our social world, one that permits us to be better able to hear and affirm stories of gender diversity in childhood and adolescence, including within health services'. The stories told in this paper confirm that parents/carers identify waiting for care as an extremely difficult experience for both children and their families, one associated with a sense of profound loss and prolonged uncertainty.

In contrast Ker et al (2020) describe how adult service users value the experience of gender affirmation accessed in a primary care setting in an Aotearoa New Zealand University. While 'time' was a key theme dominating their talk, participants described the range of benefits to accessing care in a general practice environment as including not having to wait. Importantly, the analysis is informed by frameworks which distinguish 'medicalisation' and '(de)pathologisation' to ground the argument that gender affirming care can be provided in general practice settings without perpetuating the construction of gender diversity as disorder or relying on a 'gender dysphoria' diagnosis (e.g. Johnson, 2019; Suess Schwend, 2020).

Another interpretation of our special issue theme is that trans health is itself *waiting to be seen as a legitimate field* of health care practice. Beyond the important sociological question of how medical authority is established in a 'fractured society' (Scambler, 2020), this crisis of authenticity is fuelled by the highly problematic tendency in both clinical and non-clinical contexts to question trans experience or, as Florence Ashley has so powerfully put it, 'mistrusting trans voices' (2019, p. 480). These twinned strategies of delegitimization are repeatedly observed in the external attacks on trans health, with critics deliberately casting aspersions on both the clinicians who provide gender affirming care (e.g. Watson, 2020), and trans people's capacity to determine their own health needs and to provide informed consent to access the care they desire (e.g. shuster, 2019). Even within health care settings that aim to be inclusive and supportive, trans people are still required to produce quite specific and 'sanitised' (Ashley, 2019) narratives of their experiences in order for them to be recognised as 'authentic' by clinicians (MacKinnon, Grace, Ng, Sicchia, & Ross, 2020), including familiar tropes such as 'I was always a man inside and I need my body to match' (Heyes & Latham, 2018, p. 180). As Austin H. Johnson reminds us, the resources required to deploy the required evidence in the form it is anticipated, are not 'equally available to all trans people in all contexts', and even the most well-prepared and well-resourced trans person may not be afforded 'the credibility to be positioned as an authority of one's own experiences within medicalised contexts' (2019, p. 528).

This question of how trans health is made legitimate is explored by Shepherd and Hanckel (2020, p. 41) in their analysis of how specific 'ontologies of transition' are constructed in guidelines governing trans health practice in England, contrasted with accounts from trans people themselves. Informed by Ruth Pearce's (2018) framework distinguishing 'trans as condition' from 'trans as movement', the authors argue that trans health guidelines rely on conceptualisations of medical transitions as linear and binary, which makes (in)visible the many more 'complex ways of being trans' (Latham, (2016), p. 349), including what Linander et al (2020) have described as 'the problem of (non)linear gender'.

Given the intensity of the debates about access to gender affirming care, we found it refreshing that Bartholomaeus, Riggs, and Sansfaçon (2020, p. 58) chose to focus on understanding how Australian young people, and their parents, articulate their expectations for, and experiences of, high-quality gender affirming care. Drawing on Ansara and Hegarty's (2013, p. 162) definition of cisgenderism as 'the discriminatory ideology that delegitimises people's own designations of their genders and bodies', the authors argue for a remediation of even the most subtle forms of cisgenderism, including the problematic assumption that gender affirming care should remain the purview of specialists.

This links us to our final interpretation of the special issue theme of 'waiting to be seen', which recognises that, in most contexts, trans people are still *waiting to be seen in the social structures and systems* that impact health and wellbeing, including law, policy, media and research domains. Although the public visibility of trans lives has increased in recent years, the impacts and politics of this increasing attention are complex (Koch-Rein, Haschemi Yekani, & Verlinden, 2020). For example, in Australia, while there has been a welcome focus on strengthening the collection of data on diverse genders and sexualities (Callander et al., 2019; Lyons, Anderson, Rasmussen, & Gray, 2020), including non-binary, fluid and multiple genders (Callander et al., 2020), not all participants feel safe to be openly trans in research (Vivienne, 2011). And while there is intensive work underway around the world to change the laws and policies which constrain changes to identity documentation, the visibility that comes from these efforts can also lead to increased surveillance and threats to personal and community safety (Wundram Pimentel & Leonardo Segura, 2018). In particular areas of trans health, such as paediatric and adolescent health care, protecting and sustaining the delivery of services may be considered more important than increasing the public visibility of those who are providing and accessing these services.

Speaking to this ambivalence, Albury, Dietzel, Pym, Vivienne, and Cook (2020, p. 72) argue that the strategic practices employed by Australian trans dating app users to feel safer and avoid harassment when seeking intimate connections could usefully inform the redesign of sexual health systems, many of which remain 'hard-wired' by binary understandings of genders and sexualities. Drawing on Paul B Preciado's concept of 'pharmacopornographisation' (2013), the authors argue that the forms of self-disclosure enforced by both dating apps and sexual health services – which make gender and sexuality visible in particular forms – can produce both harm *and* valued outcomes (for more on digital self-representations of gender diversity, see Vivienne, 2017).

There will be continuing rich opportunities for sociologists to contribute careful, critical and collaborative perspectives on trans health which seek to promote inclusion and reduce harm in the coming years. While the alliances between trans communities, clinicians and researchers grow stronger by the day, so too does the vehemence of those seeking to undermine this alliance through legal challenges, opinion pieces, and direct threats to the safety and dignity of trans people. In every setting that is polarised, however, there are also countless examples of respectful, collaborative work underway including in the domains of sport, education, and health (ACON, 2020; Storr, Robinson, Davies, Nicholas, & Collison, 2020), grounded in a shared understanding that the affirmation of gender diversity supports equity for all. We look forward to championing a new generation of sociological and social science research to support trans people in seeking to assert their fundamental rights, including the right to health, in every context.

Note

1. The emergence of 'trans' as a category of meaning has been widely discussed (for a brief history, see Shepherd and Hanckel in this special issue). We are using this shortened term as an umbrella concept to recognise both transgender and gender diverse people, including non-binary people, and those with fluid and multiple genders (Cover, 2019).

References

ACON. (2020, December 17). TransHub. Retrieved from https://www.transhub.org.au/

Aizura, A. Z. (2018). *Mobile subjects: Transnational imaginaries of gender reassignment.* Durham: Duke University Press.

Albury, K., Dietzel, C., Pym, T., Vivienne, S., & Cook, T. (2020). Not your unicorn: Trans dating app users' negotiations of personal safety and sexual health. *Health Sociology Review*, *30*(1), 72–86. doi:10.1080/14461242.2020.1851610

Ansara, Y. G., & Hegarty, P. (2013). Misgendering in English language contexts: Applying non-cisgenderist methods to feminist research. *International Journal of Multiple Research Approaches*, *7*(2), 160–177. doi:10.5172/mra.2013.7.2.160

Appenroth, M. N., & Varela, M. D. M. C. (Eds.). (forthcoming). *Trans health: Global perspectives on care for trans communities.* Germany: Transcript Publishing.

Ashley, F. (2019). Gatekeeping hormone replacement therapy for transgender patients is dehumanising. *Journal of Medical Ethics*, *45*(7), 480–482. doi:10.1136/medethics-2018-105293

AusPATH. (2020). *AusPATH statement on medical gender affirmation and Re Imogen.* Retrieved December 17, from https://auspath.org/advocacy/

Bartholomaeus, C., Riggs, D. W., & Sansfaçon, A. P. (2020). Expanding and improving trans affirming care in Australia: Experiences with healthcare professionals among transgender young people and their parents. *Health Sociology Review*, *30*(1), 58–71. doi:10.1080/14461242.2020.1845223

Blakey, A. G., & Treharne, G. J. (2019). Overcoming barriers to transgender healthcare education in Aotearoa New Zealand. *New Zealand Journal of Educational Studies*, *54*(2), 357–366. doi:10.1007/s40841-019-00143-2

Brosnan, C., & Kirby, E. (2016). Sociological perspectives on the politics of knowledge in health care: Introduction to themed issue. *Health Sociology Review*, *25*(2), 139–141. doi:10.1080/14461242.2016.1174055

Byron, P., Rasmussen, S., Wright Toussaint, D., Lobo, R., Robinson, K., & Paradise, B. (2017). *'You learn from each other': LGBTIQ young people's mental health help-seeking and the RAD Australia online Directory.* Abbotsford, Victoria: Young and Well Cooperative Research Centre. doi:10.1080/22041451.2015.1110085

Callander, D., Newman, C. E., Holt, M., Rosenberg, S., Duncan, D. T., Pony, M., … Cook, T. (2020). The complexities of categorizing gender: A hierarchical clustering analysis of data from the first Australian Trans & Gender Diverse Sexual Health Survey. Published online in *Transgender Health* on 30 July 2020. https://doi.org/10.1089/trgh.2020.0050

Callander, D., Wiggins, J., Rosenberg, S., Cornelisse, V., Duck-Chong, E., Holt, M., … Cook, T. (2019). *The 2018 Australian trans and gender diverse sexual health survey: Report of findings.* Sydney, Australia: The Kirby Institute, UNSW Sydney. Retrieved from https://kirby.unsw.edu.au/sites/default/files/kirby/report/ATGD-Sexual-Health-Survey-Report_2018.pdf

Cheung, A. S., Wynne, K., Erasmus, J., Murray, S., & Zajac, J. D. (2019). Position statement on the hormonal management of adult transgender and gender diverse individuals. *Medical Journal of Australia, 211*(3), 127–133. doi:10.5694/mja2.50259

Connell, R. (2021). Transgender health: On a world scale. *Health Sociology Review, 30*(1), 87–94. doi:10.1080/14461242.2020.1868899.

Cover, R. (2019). *Emergent identities: New sexualities, genders and relationships in a digital era*. Abingdon, Oxford: Routledge.

Davies, C. (2019). *The human rights Council of Australia and co-sponsor response to the special Rapporteur's report on the right of everyone to the enjoyment of the highest attainable standard of physical and mental health*. Geneva, Switzerland: 41st Human Rights Council, United Nations Human Rights Council Interactive Dialogue.

Davies, C., Robinson, K. H., Metcalf, A., Ivory, K., Mooney-Somers, J., Race, K., & Skinner, S. R. (forthcoming). Australians of diverse sexual orientations and gender identities. In K. M. T. Dune, & R. Williams (Eds.), *Culture, diversity and health in Australia: Towards culturally safe health care*. London, UK: Routledge.

Do, T. T., & Nguyen, A. T. V. (2020). 'They know better than we doctors do': Providers' preparedness for transgender healthcare in Vietnam. *Health Sociology Review, 29*(1), 92–107. doi:10.1080/14461242.2020.1715814

Heyes, C. J., & Latham, J. R. (2018). Trans surgeries and cosmetic surgeries: The politics of analogy. *TSQ: Transgender Studies Quarterly, 5*(2), 174–189. doi:10.1215/23289252-4348617

Hines, S. (2007). Transgendering care: Practices of care within transgender communities. *Critical Social Policy, 27*(4), 462–486. doi:10.1177/0261018307081808

Johnson, A. H. (2019). Rejecting, reframing, and reintroducing: Trans people's strategic engagement with the medicalisation of gender dysphoria. *Sociology of Health and Illness, 41*(3), 517–532. doi:10.1111/1467-9566.12829

Kang, M., Robards, F., Sanci, L., Steinbeck, K., Jan, S., Hawke, C., … Usherwood, T. (2018). *Access 3: Young people and the healthcare system in the digital age- final research report*. Sydney, Australia: Department of Genderal Paractice Westmead, the University of Sydney, and the Australian Centre for Public and Poulation Health Research, University of Technology. Retrieved from https://www.uts.edu.au/sites/default/files/2019-04/Access203_young20people20and20the20health20system20in20the20digital20age.pdf

Ker, A., Fraser, G., Fleming, T., Stephenson, C., da Silva Freitas, A., Carroll, R., . . . Lyons, A. C. (2020). 'A little bubble of utopia': Constructions of a primary care-based pilot clinic providing gender affirming hormone therapy. *Health Sociology Review, 30*(1), 25–40. doi:10.1080/14461242.2020.1855999

Koch, J. M., McLachlan, C. T., Victor, C. J., Westcott, J., & Yager, C. (2020). The cost of being transgender: Where socio-economic status, global health care systems, and gender identity intersect. *Psychology & Sexuality, 11*(1-2), 103–119. doi:10.1080/19419899.2019.1660705

Koch-Rein, A., Haschemi Yekani, E., & Verlinden, J. J. (2020). Representing trans: Visibility and its discontents. *European Journal of English Studies, 24*(1), 1–12. doi:10.1080/13825577.2020.1730040

Latham, J.R. (2016). Trans men's sexual narrative-practices: Introducing STS to trans and sexuality studies. *Sexualities, 19*(3), 347–368. doi:10.1177/1363460715583609

Linander, I., Lauri, M., Alm, E., & Goicolea, I. (2020). Two steps forward, one step back: A policy analysis of the Swedish guidelines for trans-specific healthcare. *Sexuality Research and Social Policy*. doi:10.1007/s13178-020-00459-5

Lupton, D. (2020). Special section on 'sociology and the coronavirus (COVID-19) Pandemic'. *Health Sociology Review, 29*(2), 111–112. doi:10.1080/14461242.2020.1790919

Lyons, A., Anderson, J., Rasmussen, M. L., & Gray, E. (2020). Toward making sexual and gender diverse populations count in Australia. *Australian Population Studies, 4*(2), 14–29.

MacKinnon, K. R., Grace, D., Ng, S. L., Sicchia, S. R., & Ross, L. E. (2020). "I don't think they thought I was ready": How pre-transition assessments create care inequities for trans people with complex mental health in Canada. *International Journal of Mental Health, 49*(1), 56–80. doi:10.1080/00207411.2019.1711328

Malatino, H. (2020). *Trans care*. Minneapolis, US: University of Minnesota Press.

Newman, C. E., Prankumar, S. K., Cover, R., Rasmussen, M. L., Marshall, D., & Aggleton, P. (2020). Inclusive health care for LGBTQ+ youth: Support, belonging, and inclusivity labour. *Critical Public Health*, doi:10.1080/09581596.2020.1725443

Newman, C., MacGibbon, J., Smith, A. K. J., Broady, T., Lupton, D., Davis, M., … Holt, M. (2020). *Understanding trust in digital health among communities affected by BBVs and STIs in Australia*. Sydney, Australia: Centre for Social Research in Health, UNSW Sydney. doi:10.26190/5f6d72f17d2b5

Pearce, R. (2018). *Understanding trans health*. Bristol: Bristol Policy Press.

Pearce, R., Erikainen, S., & Vincent, B. (2020). TERF wars: An introduction. *The Sociological Review*, *68*(4), 677–698. doi:10.1177/0038026120934713

Plummer, K. (1995). *Telling sexual stories*. London, New York: Routledge.

Preciado, P. B. (2013). *Testo junkie: Sex, drugs and biopolitics in the pharmacopornographic era*. New York: The Feminist Press.

Robinson, K. H., Bansel, P., Denson, N., Ovenden, G., & Davies, C. (2014). *Growing up queer: Issues facing young Australians who are gender variant and sexuality diverse*. Melbourne: Young and Well Cooperative Research Centre. Retrieved from http://www.youngandwellcrc.org.au/wp-content/uploads/2014/02/Robinson_2014_GrowingUpQueer.pdf

Robinson, K. H., Townley, C., Ullman, J., Denson, N., Davies, C., Bansel, P., … Lambert, S. (2020). *Advancing LGBTQ+ safety and inclusion: Understanding the lived experiences and health needs of sexuality and gender diverse people in Greater Western Sydney*. Sydney, Australia: Western Sydney University & ACON. Retrieved from https://researchdirect.westernsydney.edu.au/islandora/object/uws:58041/

Rickett, B., Johnson, K., Ingle, H., & Reynolds, M. (2020). Support for parents/carers of primary school aged gender diverse children in England, UK: A mixed-method analysis of experiences with health services. *Health Sociology Review*, *30*(1), 9–24. doi:10.1080/14461242.2020.1857656

Sbragia, J. D., & Vottero, B. (2020). Experiences of transgender men in seeking gynecological and reproductive health care: A qualitative systematic review. *JBI Evidence Synthesis*, *18*(9), 1870–1931. doi:10.11124/jbisrir-d-19-00347

Scambler, G. (2020). Covid-19 as a 'breaching experiment': Exposing the fractured society. *Health Sociology Review*, *29*(2), 140–148. doi:10.1080/14461242.2020.1784019

Scheim, A. I., Appenroth, M. N., Beckham, S. W., Goldstein, Z., Grinspan, M. C., Keatley, J. G., & Radix, A. (2019). Transgender HIV research: Nothing about us without us. *The Lancet HIV*, *6*(9), e566–e567. doi:10.1016/s2352-3018(19)30269-3

Schilt, K., & Lagos, D. (2017). The development of transgender studies in sociology. *Annual Review of Sociology*, *43*(1), 425–443. doi:10.1146/annurev-soc-060116-053348

Shepherd, A., & Hanckel, B. (2021). Ontologies of transition(s) in healthcare practice: Examining the lived experiences and representations of transgender adults transitioning in healthcare. *Health Sociology Review*, *30*(1), 41–57. doi:10.1080/14461242.2020.1854618

Shepherd, A., Hanckel, B., & Guise, A. (2019). Trans health and the risks of inappropriate curiosity published 19 September. Retrieved from https://blogs.bmj.com/bmj/2019/09/09/trans-health-and-the-risks-of-inappropriate-curiosity/

shuster, S. M. (2019). Performing informed consent in transgender medicine. *Social Science and Medicine*, *226*, 190–197. doi:10.1016/j.socscimed.2019.02.053

Storr, R., Robinson, K., Davies, C., Nicholas, L., & Collison, A. (2020). *Game to Play: Exploring the experiences and attitudes towards sport, exercise and physical activity amongst same-sex attracted and gender diverse young people*. Sydney, Australia: Western Sydney University and Twenty10 Inc GLCS NSW. doi:10.26183/5ea655c87697e

Strauss, P., Cook, A., Winter, S., Watson, V., Wright-Toussaint, D., & Lin, A. (2017). *Trans-Pathways: The mental health experiences and care pathways of trans young people - summary of results*. Perth, Australia: Telethon Kids Institute. Retrieved from https://www.telethonkids.org.au/projects/trans-pathways/

Stryker, S. D., Pallerla, H., & Pickle, S. (2020). Considerations on medical training for gender-affirming care: Motivations and perspectives. *International Journal of Transgender Health*, *21*(1), 79–88. doi:10.1080/15532739.2019.1689880

Suess Schwend, A. (2020). Trans health care from a depathologization and human rights perspective. *Public Health Reviews*, *41*(1), 3. doi:10.1186/s40985-020-0118-y

Sumerau, J. E. (2020). Expanding transgender studies in sociology. *Sociological Inquiry*, *90*(2), 217–225. doi:10.1111/soin.12345

TGEU. (2020). Transrespect versus transphobia worldwide. Retrieved December 17, from https://transrespect.org/

Treharne, G. J., Riggs, D. W., Ellis, S. J., Flett, J. A. M., & Bartholomaeus, C. (2020). Suicidality, self-harm, and their correlates among transgender and cisgender people living in Aotearoa/New Zealand or Australia. *International Journal of Transgender Health*, *21*(4), 440–454. doi:10.1080/26895269.2020.1795959

Vermeir, E., Jackson, L. A., & Marshall, E. G. (2018). Barriers to primary and emergency healthcare for trans adults. *Culture, Health and Sexuality*, *20*(2), 232–246. doi:10.1080/13691058.2017.1338757

Vincent, B. (2018). *Transgender health: A practitioner's guide to binary and non-binary trans patient care*. London: Jessica Kingsley Publishers.

Vivienne, S. (2011). Trans digital storytelling: Everyday activism, mutuble identity and the problem of visibility. *Gay and Lesbian Issues and Psychology Review*, *7*(1), 43–54.

Vivienne, S. (2017). "I will not hate myself because you cannot accept me": Problematizing empowerment and gender-diverse selfies. *Popular Communication*, *15*(2), 126–140. doi:10.1080/15405702.2016.1269906.

Watson, G. (2020). Rejection of transgender health inquiry welcomed by practitioners. *OUT in perth*. Published 7 March. Retrieved from https://www.outinperth.com/rejection-of-transgender-health-inquiry-welcomed-by-practitioners/

Winter, S., Diamond, M., Green, J., Karasic, D., Reed, T., Whittle, S., & Wylie, K. (2016). Transgender people: Health at the margins of society. *The Lancet*, *388*(10042), 390–400. doi:10.1016/S0140-6736(16)00683-8

WPATH. (2011). *Standards of care for the health of transsexual, Transgender, and gender nonconforming people (7th version)*. The World Professional Association for Transgender Health. Retrieved from https://www.wpath.org/media/cms/Documents/SOC%20v7/SOC%20V7_English.pdf

WPATH. (2020). WPATH, EPATH, USPATH, AsiaPATH, CPATH, AusPATH, PATHA Response to Bell v. Tavistock Judgment: Statement Regarding Medical Affirming Treatment including Puberty Blockers for Transgender Adolescents. Retrieved December 18, from https://www.wpath.org/policies

Wundram Pimentel, A., & Leonardo Segura, M. (2018). Paradoxes of visibility: The proposed guatemalan gender identity law. *TSQ: Transgender Studies Quarterly*, *5*(1), 83–99. doi:10.1215/23289252-4291538

Support for parents/carers of primary school aged gender diverse children in England, UK: a mixed-method analysis of experiences with health services

Bridgette Rickett, Katherine Johnson, Helen Ingle and Martel Reynolds

ABSTRACT

This paper presents findings from a UK mixed-method study that aimed to understand parents/carers' views and experiences of support received from health services for primary school age (4–11) gender diverse children and their families. Data was collected via an e-survey including 10 open-ended questions with 75 parents/carers addressing experiences with (i) primary health services, including general practice (GP) clinics and child and adolescent mental health services (CAMHS) (ii) specialist gender identity development services (GIDS) (iii) non-health related support including transgender groups and online resources. Findings are organised into four themes: 'journey to health service provision', 'view on health services used', 'waiting' and 'isolation'. Discourses about gender diversity, childhood and the validity of trans healthcare shape parental experiences, including their desire for better information, more certainty in healthcare pathways and more expedient access to support services to reduce anxiety, distress and isolation. The emotional costs of waiting are compounded by the material costs of accessing the limited number of specialist services. Experiences could be improved through ensuring GPs and CAMHS are better prepared, expanding access to trans-specific support groups for those caring for children and young people, and exploring the provision of school-based support for gender diverse primary-age children.

Introduction

In the last decade, the United Kingdom (UK), like many other high-income countries, predominantly in the global north, has witnessed a rapid rise in referrals of gender diverse[1] children and adolescents to specialist under-18s Gender Identity Development Services (GIDS) (Kaltiala et al., 2020). For example, in 2009–10 the Portman and Tavistock Clinic, the sole provider of GIDS in England and Wales, had 77 young people referred to their services. By 2017–18 (the time period in which our data was collected) this rose to 2445. The most recent figures suggest this rate is beginning to level off with referral numbers at 2590 in 2018–19 (Tavistock & Portman, 2019). In a population estimated to be 65.64 million (mid 2018), with 18.9% of that total population aged under 18 (ONS, 2018), these numbers are still very small. However, concern about the size of the annual increases in referrals, along with questions about who is being referred and how long they have to wait, has garnered unprecedented national media attention and a government inquiry (Women and Equalities Select Committee, 2016). Alongside expanding numbers, data has shown that referrals of clients who were assigned female at birth referrals were 3 times higher than for clients assigned male at birth; a significant shift since 2009. This pattern has drawn specific attention from broadsheet newspapers, the Women & Equalities Select Committee, and so-called 'gender critical' activists (Gilligan, 2019), resulting in UK public discourse currently featuring deeply inflammatory, polarised and politicised accounts of trans people's lives, identities and healthcare needs.

In the UK, this is the context in which children, young people and their families come to understand the stigma and discrimination associated with gender diverse identities and health service provision. Evidence shows that gender diverse children and their parents are most likely to access information through a range of online sources (Carlile, 2020). Their knowledge, understanding, expectation and experience of trans and non-binary identities and health service provision will inevitably be shaped by the concerns raised in these sources. In this paper, we outline in more detail the contested status of gender diversity in childhood and in the UK healthcare system, before reflecting on our empirical data documenting parent/carer expectations and experiences of accessing health care for primary school-age gender diverse children within this context.

Gender diversity in childhood: a contested possibility

There has been significant research and debate about appropriate treatment and support pathways for transgender experiences since the 1950s, but terms such as 'transgender' or 'gender dysphoria' were rarely applied to children or adolescents. UK-based education researchers have argued that transgender children have always existed, but should more accurately be categorised as 'apparent and non-apparent' in terms of their visibility within social systems (Hellen, 2009). Writing prior to the increase in numbers of children and adolescents seeking referral, Kennedy and Hellen observed that '*apparent* transgender children are relatively rare' (2010, p. 26). They argued that rather than not existing, children with these feelings chose to actively conceal them in order to achieve conformity with the heavily policed gender norms of early childhood. Despite this, trans people are very much 'aware they are transgender at much younger ages than previously considered' (Kennedy & Hellen, 2010, p. 25).

The diagnostic term 'gender identity disorder in childhood' first appeared in the Diagnostic and Statistical Manual of Mental Disorders (DSM) III in 1980, not long after the removal of 'homosexuality' in 1973. This term was initially critiqued by feminists and queer theorists (e.g. Sedgwick, 1991) for operating as a psychomedical device for normalising expressions of the cross-gender behaviour that sometimes emerged as part of a lesbian or gay identity. This argument has more recently been challenged as 'cisnormative' (Ansara & Hegarty, 2011), indicating a prejudiced ideological approach that privileges the social norm that gender expression and sex characteristics always align.

As referral rates have risen, there has also been an increased focus on confirming the validity of gender diversity classifications and treatment for those who are under 18. 'Gender incongruence in adolescence', the terminology applied by International Classification of Diseases, eleventh revision (ICD-11), has become accepted within trans healthcare as a diagnostic category that justifies access to medical support for gender affirmation (WPATH, 2012). The model of care available in the UK, like other global north countries such as U.S. and Australia, has shifted towards 'trans-affirming approaches that aim to promote gender exploration and affirmation without constraints or barriers by facilitating access to different forms of transition' (Sansfaçon, Medico, Suerich-Gulick, & Temple Newhook, 2020, p. 1). However, concerns continue to be expressed by a minority of clinical and feminist commentators about the potential risk of adverse long-term effects of hormone treatments, the strategies employed to determine informed consent to accessing gender affirming medical care among children or youth, and if so from what age those strategies should apply (e.g. Ashley, 2019; Henegan & Jefferson, 2019; Wren, 2019).

What is often overlooked in the media representations of these issues is that medical options for affirming gender among gender diverse young people, such as puberty blockers, are only one mode of support available for those aged 12–16. In line with WPATH (2012) recommendations and NHS England GIDS service specifications (NHS, 2017), full consideration of an individual's competence and capacity to consent is made during a period of careful consultation and assessment before any form of medical care is able to be accessed.[2] Access to an appropriate process of reflection is supported by evidence that only approximately 40 per cent of young people who contact the leading GIDS clinic in the UK go on to undergo physical treatments (Carmichael, 2016). Additionally, for those that do, the key purpose of 'puberty blockers' is to open up a temporal space in which the bodily transformations associated with the development of secondary sex characteristics can be paused, allowing time for further reflection about future gender pathways, while reducing the intense gender dysphoria and distress reported by these adolescents (Roen, 2011). Puberty blockers do not prevent growth or other dimensions of normal adolescent development, and so are regularly (and safely) used to delay 'precocious puberty', reduce the impacts of adolescent endometriosis or support an extended period of pre-pubertal growth among children with idiopathic short stature (Giordano and Holm, 2020).

Controversy is more apparent for the ICD-11 diagnosis 'gender incongruence of childhood', which is applied to gender diverse children who have not yet reached puberty. Many leading trans-affirmative clinicians working with gender diverse youth are against the inclusion of this diagnosis in the ICD (e.g. Winter et al., 2019). They argue that there is no need for a psychomedical framework to be applied to pre-pubescent children who are exploring their gender: 'These young children do not need puberty suppressants, masculinising or feminising hormones, or surgery. Rather, they need a safe emotional space with the freedom to explore, embrace, and express their gender identity' (Winter et al., 2019, p. 672). The need for these forms of early social support is increasing with substantial evidence demonstrating that transgender youth report higher rates of depression, suicidality and self-harm, and eating disorders when compared with their peers (Connolly, Zervos, Barone, Johnson, & Joseph, 2016; Strauss et al., 2020). Parents, advocates and transgender affirmative researchers also highlight the risk of delayed access to supportive healthcare (e.g. Carlile, 2020; Pearce, 2018), compared to evidence of the positive impact that early support with the social aspects of gender transition can have on the mental health and wellbeing of gender diverse children and adolescents (Olson, Durwood, DeMeules, & McLaughlin, 2016).

In England, the preferred route of referral to GIDS is through the local Child and Adolescent Mental Health Service (CAHMS). This is in line with WPATH (2012) guidelines that recommend that any underlying mental health concerns be explored and managed prior to progressing to the stage of accessing gender affirming care. GIDS also accept referrals through the primary care system, from a general practitioner/doctor (GP), and from other health, education and social care professionals including LGBT+ and trans-specific groups who support gender diverse young people and their families. With greater visibility of gender diversity, parents and carers have become more knowledgeable and cognisant of early indicators of gender diversity, and are seeking information, support, advice and treatment for younger aged children (Carlile & Paechter, 2018). The rapid rise in referrals has undermined GIDS ability to meet these needs in a timely way. Despite expanding service provision through NHS investment and the operation of satellite clinics in cities outside of London and Leeds, waiting times have increased from 9 to 10 months in 2015 to 2 years in 2020. The negative impacts of waiting and delay are now widely expressed in social media, by both young people and their families, in contrast with the accusation that the process does not provide sufficiently in-depth care or time for consideration before commencing clinically supported forms of care (Swerling, 2020).

There are several theories currently circulating about why we might be seeing an increase in the presentation of gender diverse young people to clinical care settings, often linked to a presumed correlation between gender identity and media representations. Research has found evidence of an association between increased media coverage of topics related to trans and gender diverse people and increasing numbers of young people presenting to gender clinics (Pang et al., 2020). Controversially, some have argued that these positive media representations are fuelling an imagined phenomenon described as 'rapid onset gender dysphoria' (Littman, 2018). Interest in this unsubstantiated theory has been driven by the distress of some parents who believe that their child (adolescent or young adult) only expressed signs of gender dysphoria after having accessed information about gender diversity online. This perspective has been robustly critiqued for its lack of scientific evidence, its association with 'transantagonistic websites', and for attempting to 'weaponise scientific-sounding language evidence' to refute research evidence that demonstrates the important benefits of supporting gender affirmation (Ashley, 2020, p. 779). An alternative interpretation is that wider access to information about trans lives enables young people to have access to the language they need to describe their experience, and the confidence to seek out health services earlier, rather than waiting for adulthood. The sociologist Plummer (1996) wrote saliently about the socio-political flow of stories, social change and the ways in which stories can be transformed from inner whispers to being articulated in wider public discourse. Following Plummer (1996), we propose that it is possible we are currently witnessing an important shift in our social world, one that permits us to be better able to hear and affirm stories of gender diversity in childhood and adolescence, including within health services.

Expectations and experiences of health services among parents/carers of gender diverse children

Parental expectations of healthcare for their gender diverse children are framed by the psychosocial discourses governing gender, sexuality and child development (Johnson, 2018). These discourses include normative assumptions about gender and sexuality expressions, which can both manifest in terms of gender variance, alongside assumptions about child developmental 'stages' or 'phases', 'neuro-plasticity and the developing brain', and associated development risks such as mental ill-health and suicidal distress (Johnson, 2015; McDermott & Roen, 2016). We and others have argued elsewhere (Johnson, 2018; Winters et al., 2018) that it is also important to understand the support needs of trans and gender diverse children within these discussions, emphasising their voices and including them from a much younger age. For primary age children this dialogue will usually happen within the parent/carer dyad.

Parental expectations will also be shaped by exposure to the polarised contemporary discourses about trans healthcare for under 18s and competing interpretations of the impact of waiting for access to care. The first position, often articulated by trans-affirmative parents of gender diverse children, is that delayed access to specialist services increases the risk of gender dysphoria having devastating impacts on a child's mental health. The opposite position, often articulated by 'gender critical' authors in the UK (e.g. Brunskell-Evans & Moore, 2017), is that access to gender affirming medical care is provided too early to young people who may regret it when they are older. The latter interpretation deliberately frames access to care as an ethical question of whether and when clinical treatment should be made available for children and adolescents. However, these issues are typically expressed using divisive and dismissive terminology e.g. 'the fabrication of the transgender child', 'the transgender experiment on children' and 'the transgender trend' (Brunskell-Evans & Moore, 2017), and make unsubstantiated associations between support for gender diverse young people and the erasure or devaluing of homosexuality, particularly lesbianism (Shrier, 2020). The gender critical approach (e.g. Stock, 2018) has gained significant populist appeal in recent years through the support of specific journalists and media platforms and particular forms of Twitter dissent aiming to discredit proposed changes to the Gender Recognition Act (GRA, 2004) as well as GIDS. The GRA review proposed improving self-identification processes for gender diverse adults by allowing birth certificates to be changed without evidence of a medical diagnosis. Critics of this proposal (Stock, 2018) argued that the proposal would lead to the erasure of cisgender women's rights and safety (see Serano, 2007; Hines, 2019 for extended discussions of the false dichotomy between transgender and feminist politics, and Zanghellini, 2020 for a review of the problematic philosophical position proposed by gender critical commentators on trans inclusion).

In contrast to debates about whether or not trans healthcare should be made available, some researchers have begun to focus on documenting experiences of trans healthcare for under 18s (Carlile, 2020). Our research builds on this by introducing an innovative focus on the experiences of parents/carers of primary school-age children. Most young people who access GIDS are in the 14–16 years old category. This is not surprising given the lengthy waiting times after a referral is secured, and because they specialise in puberty specific treatment pathways. However, GIDS also receive referrals for much younger children, reflecting an emerging need for information and support for pre-pubescent children and their families. The aim in this study was to understand the health care expectations and experiences of parents/carers seeking support for gender diverse children aged 4–12 years.

Methods and analysis

This paper forms part of a larger, mixed methods project which utilised participatory research principles to engage stakeholders and practitioners (a local Trans Network, a national charitable organisation and the England-based GIDS) in the design of the study. This paper reports findings from the first study, a mixed methods e-survey, delivered via Survey Monkey, which was completed by 75 parents/carers of gender diverse primary school-aged children in the UK. The aim was to gather both metrics and qualitative, open-text data related to primary school-aged gender diverse population parent/carer experiences and expectations of health services used. The survey design and recruitment benefitted from stakeholder and practitioner collaboration in two ways. First, it increased the validity and relevance of survey items and ensured we were asking questions that filled gaps in current practitioner and on-the-ground knowledge. Secondly, the use of public social media recruitment adverts was supplemented by recruitment through our stakeholders' networks. A limitation was that our sample may have been overly representative of parents who had contact with these stakeholder networks.

The mixed methods E-survey

The cross-sectional survey included 52 questions in 4 sections, 14 of which were open-text. First, a background and initial presentation section included six questions, e.g. 'How old is your child at the moment?' Second, an involvement with services section contained 7 questions about GP/Doctor, GIDS, Child and Adolescent Mental Health Services (CAHMS), School and Educations Services and Other services, e.g. 'Can you please give an example of how your Doctor / GP Service/ GIDS/CAMHS/ School Education was helpful?' The third section focused on overall views of services provided. Finally, we collected 10 demographic information responses about the parents/carers, the children and their families. The survey generated 86 responses. For quality purposes, only 75 survey respondents who answered 75% of key survey questions were included in the analysis.

Analytic methods

The quantitative data was summarised using SPSS software to establish frequency data for all 38 quantitative items in the E-survey. The qualitative data set was derived from the 14 open-text questions, generating 14,029 words across 441 responses, ranging from one word to 977. This data was analysed thematically by coding and identification of overarching themes about family experiences of health care service provision. Thematic Analysis is a flexible type of qualitative analysis that is useful for identifying broad patterns of meaning across a data set, including open-text survey data (Braun & Clarke, 2006).

Findings

In this section we present key descriptive statistics from the quantitative survey data including 'demographics', as well as two themes: 'journey to health service provision' and 'views of health services used'. We then outline two overarching themes generated from the qualitative open-text data, 'waiting' and 'isolation', and interpret these in relation to the literature.

Demographics

All of the respondents confirmed they were 'parents/carers'. Just 26/75 reported their gender identity, and of the 26, most identified as women (just three as men) and cisgender, and one person as a trans parent/carer. Most were 'White', except one 'mixed heritage' respondent. All were either in the 41–50 years old (50%) or the 31–40 years old (47%) age groups. The study sample was geographically distributed across Scotland, Wales and England, however no parents/carers responded from Northern Ireland. This is broadly representative of UK population estimates (Office for National Statistics, 2020), with 83.5% living in England, and the English sample scattered fairly representatively around all main regions, with the exception for the North-West and South-East which were represented at 2–3 times higher than the UK national population estimates at region level (Statistica, 2020).

The average age of the child concerned, at the time of the survey, was 8.5 years old (ranging between 4 and 12 years old). These children were equally as likely to have been assigned male or female at birth (51% presumed male, 49% presumed female). Just over half were 'currently living all the time as the gender they identify with' (53%), 13% were 'living some of the time as the gender they identified with' and 17% had not socially transitioned. Most of the gender diverse children were defined as 'White' (86%), 9% 'mixed/multiple' heritage, 2% 'Black' and 3% 'other'. The sample closely matched the national heritage profile, in addition to family household data (Office for National Statistics, 2011 Census) and reported family income (Office for National Statistics, 2018).

Journey to health service provision

Once families became aware that their child was displaying gender diverse characteristics, most (68%) indicated that they conducted online research to explore the subject, with 56% then contacting a gender support group. Most respondents (64%) reported they had discussed these observations with someone else within a month, but for a small number (16%) it took more than a year to do so. There was a 4 year gap between the average age of the child when their parent/carer became aware that they were displaying gender diverse characteristics (median age = 3 years old), and the average age of the child when parents/carers initially consulted the first of the statutory services (i.e. GP/CAMHS/GIDS.).

Views of health services used

Eighty-five percent of parents/carers had consulted their GP service about their gender diverse child (Mean age = 7 years old). Of these participants, most felt their initial concerns had been taken seriously (65%). However, only a small proportion agreed their GP was knowledgeable about the needs of primary-aged gender diverse children or their parents/carers (16%), that they had received good advice (24%), that they had received good support (38%) or that they were happy with the service (34%). While over half of the respondents (59%) reported that they had been referred on to other services, many parents/carers reported they had to often direct their GP service to appropriate resources or provide them with the specific information about where they needed the GP to refer them on to.

Mostly following a GP referral, 62% of the sample had consulted their CAMHS with the average age of first contact for their gender diverse child at 8 years old. Some parents/carers indicated (in the open-text responses) that they viewed contact with CAMHS as a necessary 'gateway' to access a referral to GIDS. Again, most (65%) agreed that CAMHS took their concerns seriously, but the vast majority disagreed with the statement that the service was knowledgeable about the needs of gender diverse children (64%) or their parents/carers (67%). As with the GP service, a lack of good advice (only 15% agreed) and lack of good support received (27% agreed) often accompanied a disagreement with the statement that CAMHS was knowledgeable about family needs.

A large proportion of families (66%) reported they had consulted a GIDS (Mean and Median age = 9 years old), nearly all using Tavistock services in England (e.g. London or Leeds), and the remainder accessing Sandyford (Scotland). Most who had not yet accessed a GIDS were on the waiting list to access one. Most respondents (76%) agreed that the GIDS clinics took their concerns seriously, but only half agreed that GIDS were knowledgeable about the needs of gender diverse children and their parents/carers (53%). Only 39% agreed that the waiting time to see the GIDS team was acceptable, and less than half (42%) were happy with the service they received. Nevertheless, most (65%) agreed they would be happy to return to the service in the future. Finally, a third of parents/carers selected a community-led group for supporting gender diverse children and their parents in the UK as the most useful form of support (32%), followed by Schools (20%), GIDS (13%), GP (8%) and CAMHS (2%).

'Waiting'

The first overarching theme in qualitative accounts of the support provided by health services for gender diverse children was the experience of waiting, which was frequently entwined with a feeling of loss. This theme was described by participants in three main ways. First, waiting was a feature at every step of the journey through healthcare and was described as unwanted and unnecessary. Second, waiting was associated with a loss of time which caused unnecessary harm to their children. Third, waiting was experienced as a feeling of being suspended in a vacuum, not knowing what to do for the best to support their child, while awaiting official information. All of these experiences created significant frustration, worry and anxiety for parents and carers, as in the following example:

> Extract 1: The waiting lists are too long, and our commute to the GIDS is two hours on a train each way. It's expensive … I lose a day's pay and have to pay £60+ in train fares … we have to stay overnight in a hotel. (Parent/Carer 38)

The parent/carer here describes the temporal and material dimensions of waiting, including the 'loss of time' involved in waiting to be seen, as well as the time spent on lengthy journeys to GIDS due to the limited geographical spread of specialist provision in the UK. The material cost of travel, accommodation and lost wages also had an impact on personal finances; an experience shared widely amongst parents and carers needing access to specialist services.

Waiting was also experienced as a vital loss of time in the development of the children for whom the participants were caring. Slow access to GIDS meant that some children had begun to experience adolescent-related physical changes associated with gender dysphoria and distress, particularly secondary sex characteristics such as breasts. For this parent/carer and many others, the degree of distress expressed by their child was keenly felt, despite finding the services helpful and useful:

> Extract 2: [GIDS] waiting list is very long (around 12 months), but they were very approachable. Still waiting for appointment. Hopefully more funding would be available to expand service. Hormone blockers would be good to be prescribed by GP as waiting lists are so long. Having well developed breasts and periods is quite a source of distress for my child. (Parent/Carer 49)

As already noted in the themes on the journey to and experiences of health services, children, young people and their families have often been living with gender diversity for a significant amount time before they family chose to seek out health service support. For those with a clear idea about the appropriate pathway for their child, the length of time spent waiting for an appointment at GIDS, followed by a further period of exploration and reflection, can feel like an unnecessary delay to achieving relief from the bodily distress created by the development of secondary sex characteristics associated with puberty. This is one of the challenges faced in navigating the current system in the UK, in which years can stretch out from the initial discussion within the family to accessing GIDS, and during that time significant changes can happen to the child as they enter puberty. Being prescribed puberty blockers is for some parents a way to put these changes on hold, described as a chance to 'pause' and reflect on the experience of gender development through adolescence (Roen, 2011). This aspect of time for reflection after having accessed GIDS was welcomed by some parents:

> Extract 3: It's giving my child time to process life and future as he is and will provide blockers to allow the extra time. (Parent/carer 56)

Many parents/carers also reported feeling that they and their child were stuck in a knowledge vacuum during long periods of waiting. This led to 'anxiety and other issues' which were perceived as being avoidable (extract 4). Here, parents felt lost and unsure without expert guidance and left to rely on 'unofficial' information found online, which was largely aimed at older trans and non-binary people:

> Extract 4: Real need for child focused literature. My child is experiencing dysphoria but has not yet decided to socially transition despite it being a year since she came out. She is reliant on YouTube based guidance for peer support and is nervous about next steps. This is causing anxiety and other issues that could be avoided if we had access to more child friendly info whilst waiting on professional intervention. (Parent/Carer 43)

We note here that feelings of uncertainty can be exacerbated by the period spent waiting for expert intervention, or for trusted information from a GP. Parents and their children may be well-versed in accessing online media and resources but raised concerns about the availability of more appropriately child-focused resources for younger age groups. The impact of this lack of official information left these parents feeling isolated and unprepared to support their children in an informed manner. In this vacuum of guidance, many referenced the information and support offered by a national UK parent support group as vital to their survival while waiting to access statutory services (see extract 5 & 8).

> Extract 5: Need more [information]- it's a lonely place being on a waiting list for 9 months, [charity name] are a saviour and should get funding (Parent/Carer 20)

'Isolation'

Linked to the theme of 'waiting', the second overarching theme related to feelings of isolation. This presented in three main ways. First, many parents/carers shared accounts of feeling lonely and cut off from other parents. Second, many experienced their journeys through the healthcare system as a solo 'fight' or 'battle'. Finally, parents/carers reported feeling isolated as a result of their own fears of being judged and misunderstood by others.

The geographic spread of families with a gender diverse child was identified in the data as contributing to feelings of isolation and challenges in meeting other parents:

> Extract 6: Can be isolating. Don't know anyone else locally parenting [a] transgender ASD (autism spectrum disorder) child. Confidentiality prevents professionals from making helpful links. Process is long and a battle to get into services for vulnerable child. No blue-print to muddle through. (Parent/Carer 51)

The coalescence of ASD and gender diversity is gaining more attention within GIDS, but this is less common within the general population. The child of the parent/carer in extract 6 has a particular set of support needs and a lack of contact with other parents/carers in a similar situation is central to their feelings of isolation, loneliness and exhaustion. For these caregivers, this sense of isolation is exacerbated by a perception that healthcare professionals could facilitate connections to other parents/carers in a similar position but are unable to do so for reasons of confidentiality, privacy or data sharing regulations. In addition, the lack of information available for parents/carers of primary-aged children (e.g. 'no blue-print') also adds to their sense that their experience is one of isolation, disorientation and combat. In extracts 7 and 8, caregivers explain their experience of having to 'battle' or 'fight' to gain access to healthcare services, largely because of a lack of knowledge about primary-aged gender diverse children at GP and CAMHS level. A sense of survival comes from seeking out information, particularly from the 'internet' (extract 7), or by getting support from a UK charity (extract 8), or GIDS (extract 8):

> Extract 7: I have had to dig my way and approach people myself and fight and pester services for appointments and come across as a pushy parent, which I am not. I think GPs should all have a person in the practice that is familiar with this subject to help guide families in the right direction. Goodness know what state we would be in if it weren't for the internet. (Parent/Carer 30)

Extract 8: Be more knowledgeable! That is all. I felt like everything came from me; if I hadn't had the support of [Charity name] / GIDS God knows where we would be now. (Parent/Carer 58)

The lack of knowledge experienced within primary care and the pressure to provide information *to* services, such as GPs, CAHMS and schools, contributed to feelings of isolation. Parents/carers also reported feeling judged as a 'pushy parent' (Extract 7) by service providers, which – given their aim was simply to access the care their children needed – contributed to feelings of stigmatisation and isolation. This was described by one parent as 'isolating, judgemental and unsupportive' (Parent/carer 55).

These experiences were so marked in the data that parents/carers often made a point of reporting when a service provider was *not* experienced as 'judgemental' (extract 9), which suggests there is much work to be done in better preparing the healthcare workforce for supporting parents and children from the first time that the issue of gender diversity is raised in consultation:

Extract 9: 20 year[s] of practising as a GP … he saw that we needed support and he wasn't judgemental. (Parent/Carer 26)

Discussion

Our findings demonstrate a desperate need for improved knowledge to better support parents/carers of gender diverse primary age children. A lack of knowledge was reported in caregiver experiences of advice seeking from GPs and CAMHS, which although not acceptable, is not particularly surprising given that the numbers of gender diverse children who seek healthcare are low from a general population perspective. However, given the pathway to GIDS generally requires a referral via CAMHS, and a referral to CAMHS requires input from the GP, a more complex picture emerges whereby it is easy to understand how some parents/carers and children may experience barriers or delays if their local GP or CAMHS were not informed or supportive. Our findings also illustrate the negative experiences of waiting, the impacts of a loss of time and money on family circumstances, the cumulative impacts of uncertainty and isolation and the significant anxiety and emotional labour involved in navigating health services that are not sufficiently prepared to support gender diverse primary-age children. In addition to the emotional costs experienced by families, it is important to note that we also observed evidence of the structural and material impacts of lengthy and expensive travel times that could discourage engagement with appropriate services among families from lower socio-economic backgrounds. The very recent change to the NHS England GIDS specifications (see footnote 2) will also lead to additional financial and time costs for parents and carers if a court judgement is required to demonstrate that medical interventions are in the 'best interests' of the child.

Waiting has been described as 'one of healthcare's core experiences' (Baraitser & Salisbury, 2020, p. 128), and indeed, these parents/carers described feeling intense distress while waiting and watching for the feared impacts that puberty was likely to have on their child's gender dysphoria and mental distress. Others described waiting to be seen at a specialist clinic with the hope of accessing essential information and possibly reduce their child's and their own anxieties. Within the context of GIDS, clinicians have reported feeling very much aware of the impact of current waiting times on young people and their families and have publicly noted that the recent levelling off of referral rates should lead to improvements. As Polly Carmichael (Tavistock & Portman, 2019) states:

> We appreciate how distressing it can be for young people and their families who are waiting to be seen … Whilst we still have a substantial waiting list, this levelling off, if sustained, should allow us to more effectively anticipate the resources required to reduce waiting times. This is positive news for the young people and families referred to the service.

We argue that this phrase 'waiting to be seen' has particular resonance for those who are trans and non-binary. What we may well be witnessing in the increased referral rates and numbers seeking support for gender diverse children is a critical moment in which trans and non-binary genders are finally 'being seen' as a legitimate experience, and one that is deserving of access to medical and social care and support, if desired. What remains problematic is an overreliance on information from online sources that are unmediated and potentially inaccurate about appropriate forms of support for pre-pubescent children. Improvement in the knowledge of GPs and CAMHS has the potential to improve health service experiences of parents and their gender diverse children in primary care. A more nuanced understanding of referral pathways using age-appropriate gender diverse support groups could also reduce pressure on GIDS.

Our sample was drawn from trans-affirmative parents/carers and demonstrated how challenging and isolating their experiences can be. They flagged a lack of knowledge in many generalist services (GP/CAMHS), of waiting for access to 'expert' knowledge in specialist service (GIDS) and chronic experiences of uncertainty, anxiety and distress. While it is understandable that parents/carers desire more certainty and reassurance in seeking the 'next steps' for their gender diverse children, focusing too much on issues of 'certainty' also risks perpetuating an overly limited narrative of medical transition or affirmation as the only or at least most familiar pathway for gender diverse children. The notion of achieving certainty regarding gender implies an either/or discourse that privileges binary assumptions about how gender is experienced. This is contra to UK and Australian school-based research that suggest young people's understanding, experience and language around gender is expanding as the social imaginary becomes ever more infused with the values and rights frameworks relating to gender equality and gender diversity (Bragg, Renold, Ringrose, & Jackson, 2018; Jones et al., 2016).

We argue, then, that what is needed for parents/carers of gender diverse primary-age children, children who are not yet ready to engage with the medical services provided by specialist clinics – even if this ends up the preferred pathway – is better and earlier access to knowledge and support. Earlier access to high quality health services which include supports of a range of kinds may help families mediate and manage anxiety, distress, loneliness, and isolation and provide a safe environment in which to explore gender, celebrate diversity and develop new ways of living with uncertainty. In a sector where the waiting lists for a specialist service are extremely long, improvements need to take place to make primary care services better prepared to provide accurate knowledge and interim supports, and for support services to be more broadly resourced and accessed in other settings, including social support groups for children and their caregivers. Well-informed GP and CAMHS services could be referring parents/carers and their young children to third-sector support groups. Indeed, our findings suggest that community-run groups for gender diverse young people and parental support groups are an effective source of knowledge and support. With appropriate funding and training, they could play a more vital role in supporting parents/carers and gender diverse children, to complement the pathways into and services provided within specialist clinical care settings. Although not explored here, schools also have an important role to play in supporting the needs of young gender diverse children and should be meaningfully engaged in the design and delivery of a more integrated and well-informed system of support services (Carlile, 2020).

Conclusion

International guidelines for advancing transgender health focus on recommendations for provision of affirmative pathways into care, with the expectation that appropriate forms of healthcare will be accessible, albeit within the constraints of local health systems and cultural practices (WPATH, 2012). Our research demonstrates that even if there is a commitment to this model of care, as there is in the UK, experiences of healthcare are shaped by material challenges within a public health system that is often overloaded and under-resourced. In our analysis of the experiences and expectations of the caregivers of gender diverse children, the issues faced in the UK context include long waiting lists, barriers to physically accessing specialist services that require significant time and travel, potentially excluding lower income families, and a referral pathway that often creates further delay because of a lack of initial knowledge and support in both primary care and CAMHS. These issues are located in a context in which the knowledge of many people about trans issues, including parents/carers and those working in generalist primary care settings, is shaped by a highly emotive and divisive public 'debate' about the legitimacy and value of trans lives. This context therefore adds in additional, and unhelpful, questions about the safety and appropriateness of trans healthcare models for under 18s and invites parental anxiety to be heightened about the issue of children and young people's right and ability to consent. The current context also features shaming discourses about the role of 'pushy parents' and implies they are motivated by a desire for 'gender normality' in their children, which is believed to be driven by a form of homophobia. In this context, it not surprising that parents describe themselves as feeling isolated and judged, struggling to find support appropriate for their children and themselves. We look forward to more positive frameworks and pathways being developed in the UK in the coming years to improve the experience of gender diverse children and their caregivers.

Note

1. We use gender diverse in this paper to recognise children's gender expressions that do not conform to socially expected norms. Gender diverse can also be referred to as gender variant, trans, non-binary and gender queer, although some of these terms are more readily associated with adolescent and adult identifications rather than primary age children.
2. As this article went to press, NHS England released new guidelines with regards to consent and the administration of puberty blockers, dramatically changing the care pathways for gender diverse young people. This change followed the findings of a High Court legal

challenge against the Tavistock Clinic. For details on new guidelines see https://www.england.nhs.uk/wp-content/uploads/2020/12/Amendment-to-Gender-Identity-Development-Service-Specification-for-Children-and-Adolescents.pdf?fbclid=IwAR1i0c2eftSQk1pxso7vogLi_pE7f7-0lxIY4rdccQdsuAUTm8EJg3-qC0M

Disclosure statement

No potential conflict of interest was reported by the author(s).

ORCID

Bridgette Rickett http://orcid.org/0000-0002-0047-9803
Katherine Johnson http://orcid.org/0000-0001-7092-4426

References

Ansara, Y. G., & Hegarty, P. (2011). Cisgenderism in psychology: Pathologising and misgendering children from 1999 to 2008. *Psychology & Sexuality*, *3*(2), 137–160. doi:10.1080/19419899.2011.576696

Ashley, F. (2019). Thinking an ethics of gender exploration: Against delaying transition for transgender and gender creative youth. *Clinical Child Psychology and Psychiatry*, *24*(2), 223–236. doi:10.1177/1359104519836462

Ashley, F. (2020). A critical commentary on 'rapid-onset gender dysphoria'. *The Sociological Review*, *68*(4), 779–799. doi:10.1177/0038026120934693

Baraitser, L., & Salisbury, L. (2020). Waiting and care in pandemic times collection [version 1; peer review: Not peer reviewed]. *Wellcome Open Research*, *5*, 128. doi:10.12688/wellcomeopenres.15971.1

Bragg, S., Renold, E., Ringrose, J., & Jackson, C. (2018). More than boy, girl, male, female': Exploring young people's views on gender diversity within and beyond school contexts. *Sex Education*, *18*(4), 420–434. doi:10.1080/14681811.2018.1439373

Braun, V., & Clarke, V. (2006). Using thematic analysis in psychology. *Qualitative Research in Psychology*, *3*(2), 77–101. doi:10.1191/1478088706qp063oa

Brunskell-Evans, H., & Moore, M. (2017). *Transgender children and young people: Born in your own body*. Cambridge: Cambridge Scholars Publishing.

Carlile, A. (2020). The experiences of transgender and non-binary children and young people and their parents in healthcare settings in England, UK: Interviews with members of a family support group. *International Journal of Transgender Health*, *21*(1), 16–32.

Carlile, A., & Paechter, C. (2018). *LGBTQI+ parented families and schools: Visibility, representation, pride*. London: Routledge.

Carmichael, P. (2016). Key issues for health services – Access to treatment, patient pathways & understanding care. Oral presentation at *Westminster social policy forum seminar: Policy priorities for transgender equality*. London, June 15.

Connolly, M. D., Zervos, M. J., Barone, C. J., Johnson, C. C., & Joseph, C. L. M. (2016). The mental health of transgender youth: Advances in understanding. *Journal of Adolescent Health*, *59*(5), 489–495. doi:10.1016/j.jadohealth.2016.06.012

Gilligan, A. (2019). Tavistock clinic reveals surge in girls switching gender, *The Sunday Times*, June 30. Retrieved from https://www.thetimes.co.uk/article/surge-in-girls-switching-gender-pwqdtd5vk

Giordano, S., & Holm, S. (2020). Is puberty delaying treatment 'experimental treatment'? *International Journal of Transgender Health*, *21*(2), 113–121. doi:10.1080/26895269.2020.1747768

GRA. (2004). *Gender Recognition Act 2004*. Available online at: http://www.opsi.gov.uk/acts/acts2004/20040007.htm.

Hellen, M. (2009). Transgender children in schools. *Liminalis: Journal for Sex/Gender Emancipation and Resistance, 81*, 99. Retrieved from https://research.gold.ac.uk/3531/1/Liminalis-2009-Hellen.pdf

Henegan, C., & Jefferson, T. (2019). Gender affirming hormones in children and adolescents 25 February 2019. *BMJ Blog*. Retrieved from https://blogs.bmj.com/bmjebmspotlight/2019/02/25/gender-affirming-hormone-in-children-and-adolescents-evidence-review/

Hines, S. (2019). The feminist frontier. *Journal of Gender Studies, 28*(2), 145–157.

Johnson, K. (2015). *Sexuality: A psychosocial manifesto*. Cambridge, UK: Polity Press.

Johnson, K. (2018). Beyond boy and girl: Gender diversity in childhood. In L. O'Dell, C. Brownlow, H. Bertilsdotter Rosqvist, & J. Du Preez (Eds.), *Different childhoods* (pp. 25–40). London: Routledge.

Jones, T., Smith, S., Ward, R., Dixon, J., Hillier, L., & Mitchell, A. (2016). School experiences of transgender and gender diverse students in Australia. *Sex Education, 16*(2), 156–171.

Kaltiala, R., Bergman, H., Carmichael, P., de Graaf, N. M., Egebjerg Rischel, K., Frisén, L., ... Waehre, A. (2020). Time trends in referrals to child and adolescent gender identity services: A study in four Nordic countries and in the UK. *Nordic Journal of Psychiatry, 74*(1), 40–44.

Kennedy, N., & Hellen, M. (2010). Transgender children: More than a theoretical challenge. *Graduate Journal of Social Science, 7*(2), 25–43.

Littman, L. (2018). Parent reports of adolescents and young adults perceived to show signs of a rapid onset of gender dysphoria. *PLoS One, 13*(8), e0202330. doi:10.1371/journal.pone.0202330

McDermott, E., & Roen, K. (2016). *Queer youth, suicide and self-harm: Troubling subjects, troubling norms*. London: Palgrave.

NHS England. (2017). *NHS standard contract for gender identity development service for children and adolescents*. Retrieved from https://www.england.nhs.uk/wp-content/uploads/2017/04/gender-development-service-children-adolescents.pdf

Office for National Statistics. (2011). *2011 census: Population and household estimates for the United Kingdom, March 2011*. Retrieved from https://www.ons.gov.uk/peoplepopulationandcommunity/populationandmigration/populationestimates/datasets/2011censuspopulationandhouseholdestimatesfortheunitedkingdom

Office for National Statistics. (2018). *Overview of the UK population: November 2018*. Retrieved from https://www.ons.gov.uk/peoplepopulationandcommunity/populationandmigration/populationestimates/articles/overviewoftheukpopulation/november2018#:~:text=The%20UK%20population%20is%20ageing,With%20ongoing%20advances&text=An%20estimated%2018.9%25%20of%20the,to%2064%20years%20in%202017

Office for National Statistics. (2020). *Population estimates for the UK, England and Wales, Scotland and Northern Ireland: mid-2019*. Retrieved from https://www.ons.gov.uk/peoplepopulationandcommunity/populationandmigration/populationestimates/bulletins/annualmidyearpopulationestimates/mid2019estimates

Olson, K. R., Durwood, L., DeMeules, M., & McLaughlin, K. A. (2016). Mental health of transgender children who are supported in their identities. *Pediatrics, 137*(3), e20153223. doi:10.1542/peds.2015-3223

Pang, K. C., de Graaf, N. M., Chew, D., Hoq, M., Keith, D. R., Carmichael, P., & Steensma, T. D. (2020). Association of media coverage of transgender and gender diverse issues with rates of referral of transgender children and adolescents to specialist gender clinics in the UK and Australia. *JAMA Network Open, 3*(7), e2011161. doi:10.1001/jamanetworkopen.2020.11161

Pearce, R. (2018). *Understanding trans health: Discourse, power and possibility*. Bristol, UK: Policy Press.

Plummer, K. (1996). *Telling sexual stories: Power, change, and social worlds*. London: Routledge.

Roen, K. (2011). The discursive and clinical production of trans youth: Gender variant youth who seek puberty suppression. *Psychology & Sexuality, 2*(1), 58–68.

Sansfaçon, A. P., Medico, D., Suerich-Gulick, F., & Temple Newhook, J. (2020). 'I knew that I wasn't cis, I knew that, but I didn't know exactly': Gender identity development, expression and affirmation in youth who access gender affirming medical care. *International Journal of Transgender Health*. doi:10.1080/26895269.2020.1756551

Sedgwick, E. K. (1991). How to bring your kids up gay. *Social Text*, *29*, 18–27.

Serano, J. (2007). *Whipping girl: A transsexual woman on sexism and the scapegoating of femininity*. New York: Seal Press.

Shrier, A. (2020). *Irreversible damage: The transgender craze seducing our daughters*. Washington, DC: Regnery Publishing.

Statistica. (2020). *Population in England in 2019, by region*. Retrieved from https://www.statista.com/statistics/294681/population-england-united-kingdom-uk-regional/

Stock, K. (2018, October 1). Why self-identification should not legally make you a woman. *The Conversation*. Retrieved from https://theconversation.com/why-self-identification-should-not-legallymake-you-a-woman-103372

Strauss, P., Cook, A., Winter, S., Watson, V., Wright Toussaint, D., & Lin, A. (2020). Associations between negative life experiences and the mental health of trans and gender diverse young people in Australia: Findings from trans pathways. *Psychological Medicine*, *50*(5), 808–817.

Swerling, G. (2020). Former transgender patient will tell court that sex change clinic is putting children on 'tortuous' path. *The Telegraph*. Retrieved from https://www.telegraph.co.uk/news/2020/01/22/former-transgender-patient-tells-court-sex-change-clinic-putting/

Tavistock, & Portman. (2019). *Referrals to the gender identity development service (GIDS) level off in 2018–19*. Retrieved from https://tavistockandportman.nhs.uk/about-us/news/stories/referrals-gender-identity-development-service-gids-level-2018-19/.

Winter, S., Ehrensaft, D., Telfer, M., T'Sjoen, G., Koh, J., Pickstone-Taylor, S., ... Karasic, D. (2019). ICD-11 and gender incongruence of childhood: A rethink is needed. *The Lancet. Child & Adolescent Health*, *3*(10), 671–673.

Winters, K., Temple Newhook, J., Pyne, J., Feder, S., Jamieson, A., Holmes, C., ... Tosh, J. (2018). Learning to listen to trans and gender diverse children: A Response to Zucker (2018) and Steensma and Cohen-Kettenis (2018). *International Journal of Transgenderism*, *19*(2), 246–250. doi:10.1080/15532739.2018.1471767

Women & Equalities Committee. (2016). *Transgender equality*. Retrieved from https://publications.parliament.uk/pa/cm201516/cmselect/cmwomeq/390/390.pdf

World Professional Association for Transgender Health: Standards of Care for the Health of Transsexual, Transgender, and Gender Non-conforming People v7. (2012). Retrieved from https://www.wpath.org/publications/soc.

Wren, B. (2019). Ethical issues arising in the provision of medical interventions for gender diverse children and adolescents. *Clinical Child Psychology and Psychiatry*, *24*(2), 203–222. doi:10.1177/1359104518822694

Zanghellini, A. (2020). Philosophy problems with the gender-critical feminist argument against trans inclusion. *Sage Open*. Retrieved from https://journals.sagepub.com/doi/pdf/10.1177/2158244020927029

'A little bubble of utopia': constructions of a primary care-based pilot clinic providing gender affirming hormone therapy

Alex Ker, Gloria Fraser, Theresa Fleming, Cathy Stephenson, Anny da Silva Freitas, Richard Carroll, Thomas K. Hamilton and Antonia C. Lyons

ABSTRACT

The provision of gender affirming hormone therapy for transgender and non-binary people is a rapidly developing area of gender affirming healthcare. While research indicates the benefits of providing gender affirming hormone therapy through interdisciplinary primary care-based models, less is known about how service users and providers construct their understandings of affirmative approaches. In this paper, we present findings from a discourse analysis of four service users' and four healthcare professionals' talk about a primary care-based pilot clinic providing gender affirming hormone therapy in Aotearoa New Zealand. Participants employed notions of pathologisation, time, and agency in their talk to construct the clinic as a personal setting which gave service users time to make their own health decisions, while constructing hospitals as impersonal with lengthy wait times. The assessment-driven nature of best practice guidelines that governed clinicians' decision-making was constructed as constraining users' agency. Findings highlight the ongoing importance of aligning gender affirming hormone therapy with other non-disease types of healthcare, and suggest new ways for achieving this through affirmative approaches to healthcare.

Many transgender and non-binary (trans) people, whose gender does not align with that presumed for them at birth, view gender affirming hormone therapy as medically necessary. Despite research demonstrating the positive effects of gender affirming hormone therapy on trans people's wellbeing (Bockting, Miner, Swinburne Romine, Hamilton, & Coleman, 2013; Hughto, Reisner, & Pachankis, 2015), many people around the world have had difficulties accessing hormones due to the lack of trained healthcare professionals (Dewey, 2015; McPhail, Rountree-James, & Whetter, 2016; Safer et al., 2016; Snelgrove, Jasudavisius, Rowe, Head, & Bauer, 2012), lengthy wait times (Clark, Veale,

Greyson, & Saewyc, 2018; Erasmus, Bagga, & Harte, 2015; Fraser, 2020) and lack of dedicated funding and clear information on how to access care (Veale et al., 2019). Such barriers are typically underpinned by dominant understandings of gender that privilege cisgender (non-trans) interpretations (Pearce, 2018). These systems, which tend to position gender affirming healthcare as elective or non-urgent (Stryker, 2008; Wi-Hongi, Grieg, & Hazenberg, 2017) are being increasingly challenged by trans health advocates who frame access to gender affirming healthcare as a human rights issue (Davy, Sørlie, & Schwend, 2018; Schwend, Winter, Chiam, Smiley, & Cabral Grinspan, 2018).

Medicalisation and (de)pathologisation

The evolving discourses about gender diversity both construct, and are constructed by, medical discourses around gender dysphoria and transitioning (Riggs et al., 2019). As such, medicalisation and (de)pathologisation are both useful concepts to assist in understanding gender affirming healthcare. Medicalisation refers to the process by which human experiences and conditions become framed as medical issues that require intervention or treatment (Illich, 1975; Szasz, 1970). Though some earlier sociologists describe medicalisation as a process of diagnosing and exerting social control (see Conrad, 1992; Zola, 1972), some scholars (e.g. Cannoot, 2019) have more recently asserted that access to healthcare should not require that a person's experience is legitimised through only being understood as a disorder or illness. This highlights the usefulness of distinguishing between medicalisation and pathologisation more closely.

In this article we draw on Sholl's (2017) distinction between medicalisation (referring to intervention and treatment) and pathologisation (relating to diagnosis and illness-related issues) to ask how gender affirming healthcare can be made accessible to trans people in medical settings, yet not reinforce the construction of gender diversity as a disorder. This is consistent with the trans depathologisation movement's efforts to ensure trans people have self-determination with regards to accessing healthcare (Sheherezade, 2017). Notably, the shift in medical discourses from narrow deficit constructions of gender dysphoria to affirmative framing of gender diversity—evident in recent revisions to the placement of and criteria for gender incongruence in the International Classification of Disorders, 11th Edition (ICD-11; World Health Organisation Europe, n.d.)—signals a need for healthcare providers to align their practice with affirmative approaches and principles of depathologisation.

Variations in gender affirming hormone therapy provision

The World Professional Association for Transgender Health's current Standards of Care, version 7 (WPATH SoC), on which Aotearoa NZ's national guidelines on gender affirming healthcare are based (Oliphant et al., 2018), are 'intended to be flexible in order to meet [trans people's] diverse health care needs' (Coleman et al., 2012, p. 2). Consequently, models of gender affirming hormone therapy differ across healthcare systems globally, depending on dominant understandings of gender, availability of resources, and healthcare providers' ability to provide gender affirming healthcare (Bonifacio, Maser, Stadelman, & Palmert, 2019; Mamoojee, Seal, & Quinton, 2017). Within the traditional diagnostic model of gender affirming hormone therapy provision, people require a formal diagnosis of gender dysphoria (American Psychiatric Association, 2013) or gender incongruence (World Health Organisation Europe, n.d.); this requirement has historically constructed and reinforced the pathologisation of trans people's experiences (Pearce, 2018; Wi-Hongi et al., 2017).

A growing number of primary healthcare services are implementing informed consent-based models to provide gender affirming hormone therapy (Cavanaugh, Hopwood, & Lambert, 2016; Schulz, 2018). In such services, primary care physicians typically work within an interdisciplinary team to offer individually tailored support to service users, and perform a mental health screening instead of a formal assessment (Bourns, 2019; Callen-Lorde, 2014; Cundill & Wiggins, 2020; Fenway Health, 2015). With sufficient provider knowledge of gender diversity, primary care settings are generally well set up to provide gender affirming hormone therapy through interdisciplinary teams (Bauer, Zong, Scheim, Hammond, & Thind, 2015; Guss et al., 2019; Wylie et al., 2016; Ziegler, Valaitis, Yost, Carter, & Risdon, 2019). An initial study of the pilot clinic on which the present study is based (Ker, Fraser, Lyons, Stephenson, & Fleming, 2020) indicated that service users were highly satisfied with the care they received in primary care. However, external understandings of medical providers as 'gatekeepers' still affected how some services users talked about their health needs with clinic staff.

The Aotearoa New Zealand context

The national healthcare system in Aotearoa New Zealand is governed by twenty district health boards, each responsible for allocating resources and funding to health services in their region (Ministry of Health, 2020). Because of this, there is no standardised pathway to accessing gender affirming healthcare across the country. The under resourcing of gender affirming healthcare in Aotearoa NZ, like in many countries, is a key determinant of unmet health needs among trans people and has created lengthy wait times for care (Fraser, 2020; Veale et al., 2019). However, there is a growing recognition of the importance of providing affirming and equitable healthcare across the country; for example, the Professional Association of Transgender Health Aotearoa (PATHA) was established in 2019 to improve healthcare for trans New Zealanders.

Gender affirming hormone therapy in Aotearoa NZ has traditionally been provided through hospital-based secondary care services (Delahunt, Denison, Sim, Bullock, & Krebs, 2018). People seeking gender affirming hormone therapy are generally required to obtain a 'readiness assessment' conducted by a qualified mental health professional in accordance with WPATH's recommendations. This assessment is usually conducted in one appointment, and the inability to provide service users with ongoing support is attributed to resource constraints. As of 2018, the growing demand for gender affirming hormone therapy in many regions meant an average wait time of one year to receive a mental health assessment through the public healthcare system (Fraser, 2020).

While some overseas studies have addressed how dominant understandings of gender and medicine affect trans people's experiences of general healthcare (e.g. Bauer et al., 2015; Hilário, 2019; Johnson, 2015a), little research has examined how gender affirming healthcare is constructed and understood by those accessing or providing gender affirming hormone therapy. The present study therefore aimed to explore how both service users and healthcare professionals constructed the pilot clinic in their talk, examining the discourses they drew on, and the implications of their constructions for understanding gender affirming hormone therapy in primary care settings. We use the term 'service users' instead of 'patients' to emphasise participants' agency in accessing care, and to resist the connotations attached to patients as unwell or passive.

Methodology

This study was informed by trans epistemology, an affirmative framework which can be used to interrogate how cisgender experiences are privileged in knowledge production (Johnson, 2015b). Accordingly, we use language and framing which acknowledge trans people as the experts in and on their own lives, rather than as 'objects and instruments of study' (Radi, 2015, p. 48). A majority of participants were trans, and the first author (who also led the present study) is trans. The study also drew on a social constructionist framework which posits that social phenomena are both constructed by the sociocultural contexts in which they are situated, and also function to construct social realities (Phillips & Hardy, 2002). The study involved in-depth individual interviews with service users and health professionals. Ethical approval was granted by the University's Human Ethics Committee.

Study location and pilot clinic

This location specific study was conducted in a clinic located in a tertiary education setting, which was established in response to growing need for gender affirming hormone therapy provision in the region to alleviate wait times in secondary care (Delahunt et al., 2018). This approach is consistent with the growing trend globally to shift gender affirming hormone therapy provision into primary care settings. Staff at a university healthcare service developed a pilot clinic in 2017 in collaboration with trans community members, students, and healthcare professionals. The clinic was supported by community organisations in the region who provide crucial support to trans community members outside of the healthcare service. As the campus-based clinic was considered one of the first of its kind in Aotearoa NZ, a small research project was conducted to gain insight to aid future provision development (see Ker, Fraser, Lyons, Stephenson, & Fleming, 2019). The pilot clinic was funded by the health service in which it was located.

The procedure within the clinic involved service users meeting with a GP to discuss the clinic process before attending an average of five counselling sessions to ensure the service user had sufficient support and information to make their decision. In an effort to enabling service users to give greater informed consent, the counsellor wrote a referral letter, and service users met with the same GP and an endocrinologist who prescribed gender affirming hormones. Although some primary healthcare providers in Aotearoa NZ are able to provide gender affirming hormone therapy without an endocrinologist present, the endocrinologist's role in this clinic was to oversee the initial appointments as the GP increased their competence in prescribing hormones. The clinic offered support between sessions, as well as after service users had been prescribed gender affirming hormone therapy. Service users who graduated or left the university were assisted by clinic staff to find a trans-friendly primary care provider. The clinic process took an average of four months from service users' initial GP appointment to starting gender affirming hormone therapy. This primary-based model adheres to Aotearoa NZ's national guidelines for providing gender affirming healthcare (Oliphant et al., 2018).

Participants and interviews

Potential participants were identified by staff at the healthcare service, including all six service users who completed the clinic at the time of the study, and four of the health professionals involved in the clinic. They were invited via email to take part in interviews about the clinic. Four service users (aged 18–26) agreed to be interviewed, two of whom were undergraduate students, and two who were taking a break from study; three defined their gender as female, and one as non-binary/neutrois. Four health professionals agreed to be interviewed; three were members of the clinic's multidisciplinary team, and one was a trans community adviser to the pilot clinic. Two health professionals were cisgender, and two were trans or non-binary. Seven participants identified as Pākehā (New Zealand European); one participant did not disclose their ethnicity. Seven participants were interviewed in person at the university, while one was interviewed by telephone. Interviews were conducted between July and September 2018 by the first author who identifies as trans. Interviews lasted between 39 and 80 min, with health professionals' interviews being slightly longer than those of service users, on average. Recordings were transcribed verbatim using a standard, basic transcription notation (from Silverman, 2001) and anonymised. All names reported here are pseudonyms.

Approach and analysis

Transcripts were analysed by the first (trans, Pākehā) and last (cisgender, Pākehā) authors, using Foucauldian discourse analysis. Discourse analysis is an approach that views language and talk as functional and achieving particular outcomes, rather than merely a neutral transmitter of information (Potter & Wetherell, 1987). Foucauldian discourse analysis similarly focuses on language, but also attends to power relations within society, and how realities are created, reinforced and sustained through dominant understandings (Willig, 2001). People employ various patterns within their talk, or coherent systems of meaning, known as discourses. Discourses may include metaphors, representations, and statements that together produce a particular meaning, or version of reality (Parker, 1990). Discourses are linked to social, historical and cultural contexts and can have connections to other discourses, all of which may construct an object in different ways (Burr, 2003). Particular discourses – or constructions in talk – can make certain ways of seeing (and being in) the world available, while closing down other ways.

Speakers draw on a number of discourses during talk, and there are often inconsistencies and contradictions between these discourses which, when identified, can provide useful analytic insight and highlight their different functions. Discourses also construct and position people in various ways, and speakers may take up or resist certain subject positions, while positioning others in other ways (Parker, 1990). Our analysis focused on identifying metaphors, phrases, grammatical features such as pronouns, and binary oppositions in participants' talk. We then identified contradictions and complexities in the patterns of meaning, which were discussed among the research team throughout the analytic process.

Findings

Participants drew on common notions of pathologisation, time, and agency to construct the clinic as an affirming process compared to the hospital system, where trans people were positioned as passive recipients of care. The clinic, however, was also constructed as inevitably constrained by the same structures apparent in the hospital system which have historically been associated with illness. This construction limited two service users' ability to discuss their mental health openly, due to concerns that existing mental health conditions may prevent or delay care. Overall, the clinic was constructed as a space in which gender affirming hormone therapy can be accessed as a necessary yet non-pathologised aspect of healthcare.

Pathologisation and power: hospital as scary, primary care as comfortable

Participants frequently drew on and resisted a discourse of pathologisation to position the clinic in opposition to secondary care models. Binary opposition is a dominant ordering principle of Eurocentric (male) thought and culture, rather than a reflection of reality (Sheets-Johnstone, 2000); although primary and secondary care are rarely delivered in binary ways, participants' dichotomising of the clinic and hospital settings was stark and functioned to position the clinic positively. Participants notably drew on similar patterns of talk through their informal and affective descriptions of therapeutic relationships and contrasted these with their formal descriptions of the hospital as a 'format' or 'procedure' associated with illness. Associating the hospital with negative affect and power imbalance functioned to conversely position gender affirming hormone therapy in a primary care-based setting as a way of normalising gender affirming healthcare.

Some participants highlighted the importance of accessing gender affirming hormone therapy in a familiar environment, constructing talk about their identity and mental health as easier with healthcare professionals with whom they had existing therapeutic relationships.

> I mean that was useful, you know, having a place I was familiar with and someone I was familiar with there, and also just being able to come up to campus and do it, it was much easier I think than- hospitals are scary! Um, than, you know, wandering through the hospital and going to the scary room and speaking to this doctor (Eli, service user)

> Going into the hospital kind of makes it seem like a bigger deal and (.) the single meeting with the hospital psychiatrist format, I think I found quite intimidating as a prospect because it's like you have this one chance to convince this person that you, that this treatment is right and you don't know [the healthcare professional] at all going in (Sam, service user)

Both Eli and Sam drew on negative affect-type terms (e.g. scary/intimidating) to describe the hospital and de-personalised terms to describe medical professionals (e.g. this doctor/this person), which constructed the hospital as an uncertain space. The familiarity of the space and the clinic staff, on the other hand, was 'useful' for Eli; others also described the clinic as useful, helpful, or supportive. These descriptions emphasise service users' agency to use the service to meet their needs, rather than having little control over being 'sent' to the hospital or proving themselves as 'trans enough' to access gender affirming healthcare.

Sam's talk about the hospital process as a 'test' alludes to a narrative commonly shared among trans communities about diagnostic models of care as gatekeeping processes (Ashley, 2019; Johnson, 2019; Pearce, 2018). Some participants resisted this dominant narrative throughout their accounts by mitigating perceived power imbalances in doctor/patient relationships, and instead drawing on a discourse of support. Michael the endocrinologist, for example, described 'this whole [clinic] process' as 'about supporting people [...] to do what they want to do, you know, it's not like other aspects of healthcare where we're gatekeeping'. A similar resistance to the clinic as a gatekeeping process was evident in Monty's (service user) account:

> [in the clinic] it was refreshing not to have to go through a gatekeeping process of saying, 'are you masculine enough or are you feminine enough?', it was simply a matter of, 'you want hormones, okay let's figure out the best way to give them to you'

Monty's use of the adjective 'refreshing' constructs the experience of not having to prove one's gender as something new or different, in contrast to the secondary care model. Further, his emphasis on collaboration in the healthcare professionals' response (i.e. 'let's figure out') positions himself and clinic staff as shared decision-makers, rather than the staff as deciding for Monty in their positions of authority.

Participants further resisted the pathologisation of gender affirming hormone therapy by positioning trans people as 'healthy'. In describing the traditional pathway of accessing gender affirming hormone therapy through the hospital, Michael (endocrinologist) shared that:

> obviously [gender affirming hormone therapy] is a very different situation altogether, we're dealing with- with um generally very healthy, generally very young individuals, y'know, who don't have diseases and we're simply supporting [them] with their healthy transition, and so we've acknowledged for a while now that this, doing this in hospital settings for that reason is not ideal.

Here, Michael's construction of healthcare professionals as supportive and the process as simpler than illness-related healthcare resists dominant constructions of gender affirming hormone therapy provision as a complex or gatekeeping process. Michael's use of the adjective 'healthy' to describe both people and their transitions alludes to a broader definition of health which includes complete social, mental and physical well-being, as well as the absence of disease (World Health Organisation, 2020 [1948]). According to this framing of health, people access healthcare for many reasons other than being 'unwell'. At the same time, Michael's association with hospital-based settings and illness suggests that the spaces in which people enter to access care, regardless of their level of health, can reinforce messages about what it means to need healthcare. These discursive manoeuvres function to locate primary care-based gender affirming hormone therapy provision as a process of resisting the historic pathologisation of trans people, which in contrast may be reinforced through requiring 'healthy' trans people to enter a space associated with illness such as the hospital. Connor, the community advisor, further resisted the pathologisation of trans people accessing healthcare:

> The advantage of having a multidisciplinary team [in the clinic] is that there's nothing wrong with us as trans people, we have got nothing wrong with us. We might have a thyroid [problem] but that's not because we're trans, we might have diabetes but it's not because we're trans, so a multidisciplinary team helps the team of health professionals stay within constructs of that person's care, not in society's views of our pathologisation.

In distinguishing someone's transness from receiving any other aspect of healthcare, Connor constructed gender affirming hormone therapy as part of a person's general healthcare as opposed to their pathologisation, a process which he frames as being 'done' to trans people. Participants frequently discussed gender affirming hormone therapy as medication distinguished from that needed to treat illnesses; this resistance to pathologising trans experiences frames gender affirming hormone therapy as a less stigmatised form of healthcare.

The importance of time when accessing gender affirming hormone therapy

Participants frequently drew on notions of time throughout their accounts in ways that constructed the clinic as quicker and with less delays than secondary care. Jordan's (service user) metaphoric description of the clinic as a 'little bubble of utopia where you can get all these appointments within a short amount of time for free' illustrates how most participants positioned the clinic as distinct from the secondary care model, which was also discussed using historical temporal markers such as 'old-fashioned' (Monty, service user) or 'behind the times' (Michael, endocrinologist). The relative timeliness of the clinic was juxtaposed with participants' perceptions of lengthy wait times for appointments in secondary care. As Monty mentioned:

> I think paradoxically even being on the [hospital] waiting list can make it worse because you're that much closer to your goal, but there's a kind of arbitrary bureaucracy standing in the way between getting you the medication that you need to continue living

Here, Monty's description of the hospital wait times as a barrier to someone's transition, further highlights how time was constructed as important to allowing people to continue with their lives, and not be in the limbo being on 'the waiting list'. Time in the hospital system was constructed as an exercise of power or a structural barrier, whereas having the time to 'just talk things through', as Monty also mentioned, suggests that time can be seen as a resource which can be used to support service users achieve their transition goals. Monty discussed the goal of the medication as enabling trans people 'to continue living', similar to Jordan's desire to 'get on' with their life, reinforcing minimal wait times as critical.

In contrast to waiting months for care, most participants described time throughout the clinic both metaphorically as a 'luxury' (Sarah, GP), and practically as 'having constant kind of contact through the [clinic] process and someone to talk to about anything I wanted to talk about' (Sam, service user). Many participants highlighted the variability of service users' health needs and the points they were at in their transitions, which served to reinforce the importance of building relationships with clinic staff over time. Constructing the clinic as having faster or 'smoother' timeframes allowed time service users to position themselves as having a 'long lovely relationship building with the clinician as well, so it's not a one-off assessment with someone that you don't know' (Sarah, GP). Sarah's juxtaposition between constructions of the 'long' clinic time and 'one-off' assessment in the hospital, further reinforces the hospital/clinic binary and importance of familiarity and certainty in gender affirming care.

This temporal construction of longitudinal support was further emphasised in Eli's account that, even after finishing the clinic, '[I] still feel like that support's there and you know, I still feel like I'm part of the system', rather than 'this medical thing that you go through and they spit you out and you've got your pills, and that's it'. Eli's vivid contrast, and a system 'spitting' service users out, constructs the hospital process as impersonal with an abrupt end-point, and unable to provide the type of ongoing holistic support available through the clinic. Because having time in healthcare interactions is often considered rare due to limited resources, this feature of the clinic was presented as enabling service users and healthcare providers to build trust. In this way, the value of time was used to resist the dominant narrative of mistrust between healthcare professionals and trans people in healthcare encounters (Lambrou et al., 2020).

Participants' extended use of journey and movement metaphors further worked to construct the clinic as an exploratory process which acknowledged the time service users had spent considering gender affirming hormone therapy prior to entering the clinic. Sarah (GP) explained that:

> I think quite often there is a really long journey before people actually get into the doctor's room and say, 'I'd like to start some hormone therapy now', and it's not a week, you know, it has sometimes been years and years and years to get to that point

Sarah and Joella similarly emphasised the work trans people had done exploring their gender or attempting to access healthcare services. This discourse of time enabled participants to account for the contradictions between service users wanting time to talk about the complexities of their identity with the counsellor, while at the same time discussing the urgency of gender affirming hormone therapy, or needing it 'ASAP for [a person's] own peace of mind' (Monty, service user). Employing the metaphor of a journey further positioned service users as capable of directing their own care throughout the clinic. Joella spoke about their role as a counsellor to keep service users in 'the driver's seat' throughout the sessions, while Sarah positioned healthcare professionals as 'pointing [trans people] in the right direction'. The participants' use of the journey metaphor constructed service users as agents, but agents who were still needing some direction, which functions to shift the healthcare professional from 'expert' to 'guide'. This has implications for how participants view power relations in healthcare settings, in which service users are traditionally considered passive recipients of care.

Bureaucracy, assessments and agency

While participants predominantly constructed the clinic as a unique and person-centred process, it was somewhat contradictorily also constructed as part of a wider medical system. Guidelines around obtaining a mental health assessment, and external constructions of accessing gender affirming hormone therapy as a gatekeeping process, functioned to limit both clinic staff and service users' agency. Most participants discussed how the pilot clinic sought to de-centre assessment from the informed consent process and positioned clinic staff as 'supporters' rather than 'assessors'. However, some participants described the requirements which clinic staff adhered to as counteracting services users' agency to determine the support they needed throughout the clinic process. The tension between the 'structural impositions' (Jordan, service user) constructed as part of an otherwise flexible pilot clinic was evident through the way participants discussed the assessment aspect of the counselling process. Most participants positioned the counsellor as an ally to service users, yet constrained by the requirement to assess service users' readiness:

> it felt like there was a procedural requirement that I got through a lot of stuff with [the counsellor] so [they] could fill in lots of paperwork and write a big letter and things, which all of which seemed excessive because [they] seemed to recognise- [they] seemed to basically be confident that in what I needed and things early on (Jordan, service user)

> there has been a tension sometimes between doing the clinical assessment, which is required-which the need for a clinical assessment, I hope one day will change, and actually just doing what might be deemed as counselling work which is attending to what the client wishes to bring (Joella, counsellor)

Here, Jordan and Joella both constructed the required assessment or readiness letter as distinct from counselling driven by service users' wishes, which participants discussed as a more valuable aspect of the clinic. Jordan framed the paperwork as serving the 'procedural requirement' rather than benefitting her as a service user, and positioned the counsellor as personally believing her needs. This constructs the perceived requirements as constraining for both the healthcare professional and service user. As shown above, Joella distanced themself from the clinical discourse they initially drew on by emphasising its requirement within the current system, and their desire for it to change 'one day'. This enabled them to prioritise the clients' needs and align herself with the counselling process, affirming service users' agency. As a member of the rainbow community themself, Joella frequently drew on trans-affirmative discourses to critique the cisnormativity of assessment-driven aspects of accessing gender affirming hormone therapy. Sam (service user) reproduced Joella's positioning in her account:

> [The counsellor] always emphasised that [they] thought the process was over-medicalised and that it shouldn't be treated as a disorder, which was nice since it had bothered me that it was treated as a disorder and I think going through the hospital [...] without that sense that the people um, there, understood the process in the same way that I did, it would have been a lot harder.

Here, Sam used Joella's statement against the pathologisation of gender dysphoria to construct her own preference of the clinic over the hospital; this shared resistance and allyship implies that Sam found it easier to access care through the pilot clinic. Sam also constructed Joella's role as a mental health professional as representing a wider system which was seen to limit Sam's ability to get the support she needed at the time:

> I did feel some pressure to pretend that my mental health was better than it was [...] because I knew that, um, they weren't meant to prescribe hormones to people who were potentially um suicidal or inclined to self-harm [...] I don't know what one could do about that, I do feel like the system as it is encourages people to lie and so not get access to the support that they need

Sam constructed the pressure to 'pretend' as due to 'the system', a generalised term referring to the clinical requirements for providing gender affirming hormone therapy that govern clinicians' actions. This enabled Sam to deflect blame from individual clinicians. Similarly, Jordan constructed her knowledge of other trans people's experiences of care as informing her views of the clinic as a gatekeeping process, stating that throughout the clinic process 'I was thinking carefully about my words [...] just to not slip up and say something that would lock me out'. Her reference to being locked out was indirectly attributed to the gatekeeping within a wider system, which functions to create this as an issue that sits outside service users' and healthcare professionals' control.

Constructing the clinic as part of a gatekeeping process contradicts Eli and Monty's (service users) accounts of the clinic as a space which people can talk openly about their transitions and mental health. Michael (endocrinologist) acknowledged but resisted this gatekeeping construction, describing service users as 'being a little bit worried that we're acting as a gatekeeping service, and that we're going to come along and say "no you can't do this" and all that sort of stuff, which isn't the case at all'. Michael's resistance to the service as gatekeeping further works to mitigate the perceived power imbalance between service users and healthcare professionals, and positions gatekeeping as more of a perception than a reality when accessing gender affirming hormone therapy.

Discussion

This location-specific study provides insight into how trans people and healthcare professionals draw on notions of pathologisation, time, and agency to frame gender affirming hormone therapy as normalised and necessary healthcare. Participants' constructions of the campus-based clinic supports the view that primary care settings which provide affirming and high-standard care can be emotionally, temporally, and physically accessible for many trans people. Providing gender affirming hormone therapy through primary care can destigmatise gender affirming healthcare as it challenges the idea that trans people make up an 'exceptional subgroup' needing specialised care (Snelgrove et al., 2012, p. 10) or hospital services (Guss et al., 2019). Over time, the growing shift towards primary care-based models of care may effect discursive shifts in the ways in which people understand trans health, considering that diagnostic models of care have historically reinforced transnormativity, or a particular way of being trans (Ashley, 2019; Davy, 2010; Johnson, 2019; Vipond, 2015).

Although there is consensus that primary care settings are generally accessible, there is ongoing debate about the requirement for a formal mental health assessment or diagnosis to access gender affirming hormone therapy (e.g. Ashley, 2019; Saad, Blackshaw, & Rodger, 2019). Participants' dual construction of the clinic process as a flexible space to talk things through which was also at times constrained by external knowledge of assessment requirements, highlights the significant challenge that providing affirmative services within an assessment-driven healthcare context represents, and the need to accommodate for trans people's varying mental health support wishes. To centre trans people's agency, healthcare providers could consider how their framing of mental health services involved in gender affirming hormone therapy informs how trans people perceive the service, and thus the information they share with healthcare professionals.

Though participants strongly resisted pathologisation, they used medicalised language to legitimise trans people's need for gender affirming hormone therapy. Similar tensions between drawing on and resisting medicalised and diagnostic discourses in trans health have been documented elsewhere (e.g. Johnson, 2019), however the nuanced distinctions between medicalisation and pathologisation could be further explored in future sociological research on gender affirming healthcare. Our findings build on Sholl's (2017) distinction between pathologisation and medicalisation which suggests that medicalised processes can occur in non-stigmatising ways. As Cannoot (2019) notes, 'fully depathologising medical transition pathways does not necessarily contradict the legitimate wish of some trans* persons to have access to trans*-specific forms of health care' (p. 4). This distinction demonstrates the potential for gender affirming hormone therapy to be situated within a medical context, yet not require a diagnosis or one-off assessment limiting service users' agency, similar to other types of healthcare such as fertility preservation. As GPs' competence in gender affirming healthcare increases, gender affirming hormone therapy will likely become more readily available in primary care-based settings without the need for hospital based care. Crucially, this requires healthcare providers to be knowledgeable about trans people's health needs and experiences, to provide affirming healthcare and avoid stigmatising trans people.

Our findings reflect a small and relatively homogenous sample of mainly Pākehā (New Zealand European) participants, including service users who were students attending a predominantly Pākehā institution with access to subsidised or free healthcare and who had previously accessed the student health service. Considering that three out of four service users were transfeminine people, the discourses they drew on may have been informed by the compounding discrimination trans women experience such as transmisogyny (Serano, 2016). Different discourses and constructions are likely to arise in other groups, such as Indigenous and people of colour, disabled, older, lower-income, or rurally located trans people, or those who have migrated from other settings, such as in Asia and the Pacific (e.g. Do & Nguyen, 2020). These findings are not intended to be generalisable, but rather indicate the prevalent discourses available to a particular demographic within a tertiary education health setting.

Despite its limitations, this study contributes relevant knowledge to a growing body of literature on gender affirming hormone therapy and its unique positioning in healthcare. Findings highlight the tensions some affirmative healthcare professionals still face due to existing discourses of trans pathologisation. Depathologising gender affirming healthcare therefore benefits from a deeper understanding of how dominant narratives of trans healthcare, such as gatekeeping and one-off assessments as 'tests', inform the provision and access to gender affirming healthcare. There is a need for consistent, collaborative approaches to providing gender affirming hormone therapy which also respond to trans people's diverse healthcare needs. As standards and models of care develop globally, it will be crucial for healthcare providers to acknowledge the ways in which existing and emerging discourses of healthcare inform service users' agency and access to equitable and affirmative healthcare.

Acknowledgements

The authors thank participants for sharing their experiences, the Sex and Gender Diverse Working Group and Mauri Ora staff who were involved in the pilot clinic, students who gave feedback on the clinic, Jemima Bullock, NGOs who support gender diverse communities in Aotearoa NZ, and the anonymous reviewers for feedback on earlier drafts. We also thank the Faculty of Health at Victoria University of Wellington for funding a research position for this study.

Disclosure statement

No potential conflict of interest was reported by the author(s).

ORCID

Gloria Fraser http://orcid.org/0000-0002-7696-7280

References

American Psychiatric Association. (2013). *Diagnostic and statistical manual of mental disorders* (5th ed.). Washington D.C.: American Psychiatric Association.

Ashley, F. (2019). Gatekeeping hormone replacement therapy for transgender patients is dehumanising. *Journal of Medical Ethics*, *45*(7), 480–482.

Bauer, G. R., Zong, X., Scheim, A. I., Hammond, R., & Thind, A. (2015). Factors impacting transgender patients' discomfort with their family physicians: A respondent-driven sampling survey. *PLoS ONE*, *10*(12), 1–16.

Bockting, W. O., Miner, M. H., Swinburne Romine, R. E., Hamilton, A., & Coleman, E. (2013). Stigma, mental health, and resilience in an online sample of the US transgender population. *American Journal of Public Health*, *103*(5), 943–951.

Bonifacio, J. H., Maser, C., Stadelman, K., & Palmert, M. (2019). Management of gender dysphoria in adolescents in primary care. *Canadian Medical Association Journal*, *191*(3), E69–E75.

Bourns, A. (2019). *Guidelines and protocols for comprehensive primary health care for trans clients.* Toronto: Sherbourne Health Centre. Retrieved from https://www.rainbowhealthontario.ca/resources/4th-edition-sherbournes-guidelines-for-gender affirming-primary-care-with-trans-and-non-binary-patients.

Burr, V. (2003). *An introduction to social constructionism* (2nd ed.). London, England: Routledge.

Callen-Lorde Community Health Centre. (2014). *Callen-Lorde Protocols for the provision of hormone therapy* . New York. Retrieved from https://callen-lorde.org/transhealth/callen-lorde-tgnc-hormone-therapy-protocols/.

Cannoot, P. (2019). '#WontBeErased': The effects of (de)pathologisation and (de)medicalisation on the legal capacity of trans* persons. *International Journal of Law and Psychiatry*, *66*, 101478.

Cavanaugh, T., Hopwood, R., & Lambert, C. (2016). Informed consent in the medical care of transgender and gender-nonconforming patients. *AMA Journal of Ethics*, *18*(11), 1147–1155.

Clark, B. A., Veale, J. F., Greyson, D., & Saewyc, E. (2018). Primary care access and foregone care: A survey of transgender adolescents and young adults. *Family Practice*, *35*(3), 302–306.

Coleman, E., Bockting, W., Botzer, M., Cohen-Kettenis, P., DeCuypere, G., Feldman, J., & Monstrey, S. (2012). Standards of care for the health of transsexual, transgender, and gender-nonconforming people, version 7. *International Journal of Transgenderism*, *13*(4), 165–232.

Conrad, P. (1992). Medicalization and social control. *Annual Review of Sociology*, *18*(1), 209–232.

Cundill, P., & Wiggins, J. (2020). *Protocols for the initiation of hormone therapy for trans and gender diverse patients.* Melbourne: Equinox Gender Diverse Health Centre. Retrieved from https://equinox.org.au/resources/.

Davy, Z. (2010). Transsexual agents: Negotiating authenticity and embodiment within the UK's medicolegal system. In S. Hines & T. Sanger (Eds.), *Transgender identities: Towards a social analysis of gender diversity* (pp. 120–126). New York: Routledge.

Davy, Z., Sørlie, A., & Schwend, A. S. (2018). Democratising diagnoses? The role of the depathologisation perspective in constructing corporeal trans citizenship. *Critical Social Policy*, *38*(1), 13–34.

Delahunt, J. W., Denison, H. J., Sim, D. A., Bullock, J. J., & Krebs, J. D. (2018). Increasing rates of people identifying as transgender presenting to endocrine services in the Wellington region. *New Zealand Medical Journal*, *131*(1468), 33–42.

Dewey, J. M. (2015). Challenges of implementing collaborative models of decision making with trans-identified patients. *Health Expectations*, *18*(5), 1508–1518.

Do, T. T., & Nguyen, A. T. V. (2020). 'They know better than we doctors do': Providers' preparedness for transgender healthcare in Vietnam. *Health Sociology Review*, *29*(1), 92–107.

Erasmus, J., Bagga, H., & Harte, F. (2015). Assessing patient satisfaction with a multidisciplinary gender dysphoria clinic in Melbourne. *Australasian Psychiatry*, *23*(2), 158–162.

Fenway Health. (2015). *Gender affirming hormone therapy for adults: Information on hormone therapy for adults age 18 and over using an informed consent model of integrated care.* Boston, MA. Retrieved from https://fenwayhealth.org/care/medical/transgender-health/.

Fraser, G. (2020). *Rainbow experiences of accessing mental health support in Aotearoa New Zealand: A Community-based Mixed Methods Study.* Dissertation. Victoria University of Wellington.

Guss, C. E., Woolverton, G. A., Borus, J., Austin, S. B., Reisner, S. L., & Katz-Wise, S. L. (2019). Transgender Adolescents' experiences in primary care: A qualitative study. *Journal of Adolescent Health*, *65*(3), 344–349.

Hilário, A. P. (2019). (Re) making gender in the clinical context: A look at how ideologies shape the medical construction of gender dysphoria in Portugal. *Social Theory and Health*, *17*(4), 463–480.

Hughto, J. M. W., Reisner, S. L., & Pachankis, J. E. (2015). Transgender stigma and health: A critical review of stigma determinants, mechanisms, and interventions. *Social Science and Medicine*, *147*, 222–231.

Illich, I. (1975). *Limits to medicine - medical nemesis: The exploration of health.* Middlesex: Penguin.

Johnson, A. H. (2015a). Normative accountability: How the medical model influences transgender identities and experiences. *Sociology Compass*, *9*(9), 803–813.

Johnson, A. H. (2015b). Beyond inclusion: Thinking towards a Transfeminist methodology. *Advances in Gender Research*, *20*, 21–41.

Johnson, A. H. (2019). Rejecting, reframing, and reintroducing: Trans people's strategic engagement with the medicalisation of gender dysphoria. *Sociology of Health & Illness*, *41*(3), 517–532.

Ker, A., Fraser, G., Lyons, A., Stephenson, C., & Fleming, T. (2019). The Trans-affirmative Healthcare Pilot Clinic (report). Retrieved from https://www.wgtn.ac.nz/health/research/trans-affirmative-healthcare-pilot-clinic.

Ker, A., Fraser, G., Lyons, A., Stephenson, C., & Fleming, T. (2020). Providing gender affirming hormone therapy through primary care: Service users' and health professionals' experiences of a pilot clinic. *Journal of Primary Health Care*, *12*, 72–78.

Lambrou, N. H., Cochran, K. M., Everhart, S., Flatt, J. D., Zuelsdorff, M., O'Hara, J. B., … Gleason, C. E. (2020). Learning from transmasculine experiences with health care: Tangible inlets for reducing health disparities through patient–provider relationships. *Transgender Health*, *5*(1), 18–32.

Mamoojee, Y., Seal, L. J., & Quinton, R. (2017). Transgender hormone therapy: Understanding international variation in practice. *The Lancet Diabetes & Endocrinology*, *5*(4), 243–246.

McPhail, D., Rountree-James, M., & Whetter, I. (2016). Addressing gaps in physician knowledge regarding transgender health and healthcare through medical education. *Canadian Medical Education Journal*, *7*(2), e70.

Ministry of Health. (2020, Feb 12). District Health Boards. Retrieved from https://www.health.govt.nz/new-zealand-health-system/key-health-sector-organisations-and-people/district-health-boards.

Oliphant, J., Veale, J., Macdonald, J., Carroll, R., Johnson, R., Harte, M., … Bullock, J. (2018). *Guidelines for gender affirming healthcare for gender diverse and transgender children, young people and adults in Aotearoa New Zealand.* Hamilton: University of Waikato. Retrieved from https://researchcommons.waikato.ac.nz/handle/10289/12160.

Parker, I. (1990). Discourse: Definitions and contradictions. *Philosophical Psychology, 2*, 189–204.

Pearce, R. (2018). *Understanding trans health.* Bristol, UK: Policy Press.

Phillips, N., & Hardy, C. (2002). *Discourse analysis: Investigating processes of social construction (Vol. 50).* London: Sage Publications.

Potter, J., & Wetherell, M. (1987). *Discourse and social psychology: Beyond attitudes and behaviour.* London: Sage Publications.

Radi, B. (2015). On trans* epistemology. *Transgender Studies Quarterly, 6*(1), 43–63.

Riggs, D. W., Pearce, R., Pfeffer, C. A., Hines, S., White, F., & Ruspini, E. (2019). Transnormativity in the psy disciplines: Constructing pathology in the diagnostic and statistical manual of mental disorders and standards of care. *American Psychologist, 74*(8), 912.

Saad, T. C., Blackshaw, B. P., & Rodger, D. (2019). Hormone replacement therapy: Informed consent without assessment? *Journal of Medical Ethics, 45*(12), 824–825.

Safer, J. D., Coleman, E., Feldman, J., Garofalo, R., Hembree, W., Radix, A., & Sevelius, J. (2016). Barriers to health care for transgender individuals. *Current Opinion in Endocrinology, Diabetes, and Obesity, 23*(2), 168.

Schulz, S. L. (2018). The informed consent model of transgender care: An alternative to the diagnosis of gender dysphoria. *Journal of Humanistic Psychology, 58*(1), 72–92.

Schwend, A. S., Winter, S., Chiam, Z., Smiley, A., & Cabral Grinspan, M. (2018). Depathologising gender diversity in childhood in the process of ICD revision and reform. *Global Public Health, 13*(11), 1585–1598.

Serano, J. (2016). *Whipping girl: A transsexual woman on sexism and the scapegoating of femininity.* Berkeley, CA: Seal Press.

Sheets-Johnstone, M. (2000). Binary opposition as an ordering principle of (male?) human thought. In L. Fisher & L. Embree (Eds.), *Feminist Phenomenology* (pp. 173–194). Dordrecht: Springer.

Sheherezade, K. (2017). *Gender is not an illness: How pathologizing trans people violates international human rights law.* GATE. Retrieved from https://gate.ngo/gender-is-not-an-illness.

Sholl, J. (2017). The muddle of medicalization: Pathologizing or medicalizing? *Theoretical Medicine and Bioethics, 38*(4), 265–278.

Silverman, D. (2001). *Interpreting qualitative data: Methods of analysing talk, text and interaction* (2nd Ed.). London, England: Sage Publications.

Snelgrove, J. W., Jasudavisius, A. M., Rowe, B. W., Head, E. M., & Bauer, G. R. (2012). "Completely out-at-sea" with "two-gender medicine": A qualitative analysis of physician-side barriers to providing healthcare for transgender patients. *BMC Health Services Research, 12*(1), 110.

Stryker, S. (2008). *Transgender History.* Berkley, CA: Seal Press.

Szasz, T. (1970). *Manufacture of madness: A comparative study of the inquisition and the mental health movement.* New York: Harper Colophon.

Veale, J., Byrne, J., Tan, K., Guy, S., Yee, A., Nopera, T., & Bentham, R. (2019). Counting Ourselves: The health and wellbeing of trans and non-binary people in Aotearoa New Zealand. Transgender Health Research Lab, University of Waikato: Hamilton NZ. Retrieved from https://countingourselves.nz/.

Vipond, E. (2015). Resisting transnormativity: Challenging the medicalization and regulation of trans bodies. *Theory in Action, 8*, 21–44.

Wi-Hongi, A., Grieg, A., & Hazenberg, E. (2017). *Towards a model of informed consent: Trans healthcare in Aotearoa New Zealand.* In M. Meyerhoff, & E. Hazenberg (Eds.), *Representing trans* (pp. 153–170). Wellington: Victoria University Press.

Willig, C. (2001). *Introducing qualitative research in Psychology: Adventures in theory and method.* Buckingham, UK: Open University Press.

World Health Organization. (2020 [1948]). Constitution of the World Health Organization. Retrieved from https://www.who.int/about/who-we-are/constitution.

World Health Organization Europe. (n.d.). WHO/Europe brief—transgender health in the context of ICD-11. Retrieved from https://www.euro.who.int/en/health-topics/health-determinants/gender/gender-definitions/whoeurope-brief-transgender-health-in-the-context-of-icd-11.

Wylie, K., Knudson, G., Khan, S. I., Bonierbale, M., Watanyusakul, S., & Baral, S. (2016). Serving transgender people: Clinical care considerations and service delivery models in transgender health. *The Lancet, 388*(10042), 401–411.

Ziegler, E., Valaitis, R., Yost, J., Carter, N., & Risdon, C. (2019). "Primary care is primary care": Use of Normalization process Theory to explore the implementation of primary care services for transgender individuals in Ontario. *PLoS ONE, 14*(4), e0215873.

Zola, I. K. (1972). Medicine as an institution of social control. *Sociological Review, 20*(4), 487–504.

Ontologies of transition(s) in healthcare practice: examining the lived experiences and representations of transgender adults transitioning in healthcare

Adam Shepherd and Benjamin Hanckel

ABSTRACT

In this article, we examine the ways transitions are constructed and represented within healthcare settings vis-à-vis lived experiences. Drawing on in-depth interviews with transgender people and data from a document analysis, we examine how transgender peoples' experiences fit within conceptualisations of transition(s) in healthcare guidance documents used in England. We take up Pearce's ([2018]. *Understanding trans health*. Bristol: Policy Press) suggestion to (re)think trans beyond 'condition', and rather as 'movement', to view being trans as a social identity rather than a defect. Our findings show how trans people and transitions are imagined through often linear narratives of movement in/out of transition. Through this framing, fluidity and gender liminal spaces are made invisible, where health care is imagined for certain transitions but not others. Our analysis attends to tensions that emerge in the complexity of transition(s) as well as the intricate ways in which transgender people are responding to often restrictive ontologies of medical transition. As a conceptual tool, 'trans as movement' can be used to create space for more expansive ontologies of gender that confront the harms and restrictions imposed by the gender binary, and offer alternative ways of (re)imagining multiplicity in transition trajectories and futures for both those in healthcare delivery, and for trans patients.

Introduction

Transitioning (also known as 'gender affirmation') involves the social and/or medical processes of altering one's expression and/or physical attributes to better align with one's gender identity, with trans healthcare commonly constructed around, and limited to, transition-related medical care (Pearce, 2018, p. 90). The health needs of transgender people, however, reach beyond their transitions. Failure to recognise this contributes to the heightened health inequalities experienced by trans individuals (Bauer et al., 2009; Lombardi, 2001; Toze, 2020). Reframing possibilities for being trans as well as for transitioning (referred to hereafter as 'trans(ition)' to describe how both trans identities and transitions are represented) in and outside of medical context contexts can provide new conceptual models to enable medicine to take account of these wider requirements for healthcare.

As Schilt and Lagos (2017) contend, there has been a shift in the approach of sociology to studying transgender people since the 1980s 'from gender deviance to gender difference' (p. 430), where whereby sociological studies now focus on the lived experiences of the diversity of gender identities and practices within everyday life. The intersections of sociology, gender studies, and queer theory have opened up 'space for alternatives to a single transgender formation (forged dialectically with the medico-legal regimes that controlled our treatments)' (Rubin, 1999, p. 190). Empirical work examining lived experience is thus not only called for, it is crucial to account for and attend to complex historically and socially situated transgender lived experiences in context (Sumerau, 2020, p. 218).

Our interest in this paper is in understanding how lived experiences of transition get (re)framed in healthcare, and the ontologies of transition that enable health care (im)possibilities. Whilst we acknowledge that not all trans people will pursue medical transitions (Davy & Toze, 2018), this study is specifically interested in the intersections of the transitioning process with medicine. As Latham (2019, p. 15) argues, drawing on Law and Benschop's (1997) work on ontology, medical representations of trans health care 'literally controls physical transformations' and 'these representations make certain ontologies impossible, even unthinkable'. Taking lived experiences and ontologies of transition in health as our object of inquiry, we draw on Ruth Pearce's (2018) framing of 'trans as condition' and 'trans as movement' to explore data from a document analysis of healthcare guidance in England along with in-depth interviews with transgender people to show how ontologies of transition have shifted in healthcare discourse(s) but often remain mis/aligned with healthcare experiences. Using and extending Pearce's framework, our findings show moments and ontologies of transition that remain outside of the purview of healthcare practice. We examine the tensions that emerge in the (im)possibilities of trans(ition) created through the documents and consider the implications this has for understanding trans health for the future.

Trans medicalised history

As Foucault (1978) argued, people are constituted through discourse, which constructs what can be thought about, and embodies and creates meaning about what is normal/abnormal, in ways that are tied to the maintenance of power. Until 1923, homosexuality and 'transsexualism' were conflated in sexological research, and people expressing such gender and sexual 'deviances' were treated as delusional and deranged (Drescher, 2010; Lev, 2013; Pearce, 2018, pp. 21–26). This gave rise to the medicalisation and pathologisation of transgender identities, with theories supporting medical interventions such as psychotherapy, which was seen as a 'cure' for trans people (Drescher, 2010; Lev, 2013). This focus on trans as curable continued to be a widely held medical belief until 1980, when 'gender identity disorder' was included as a diagnosis in the Diagnostic and Statistical Manual of Mental Disorders III (Lev, 2013). This shift also provided greater support for the emergence of 'medical transitioning', which became increasingly accepted and legitimatised within the medical community, particularly following the formation of the World Professional Association of Transgender Health (WPATH), and their publication of the International Standards of Care in 1979 (Drescher, 2010). Whilst this led to an apparent shift, from trans people being viewed as pathological and in need of a cure, to a 'normal' state of being, 'transsexualism' was not removed from the International Classification of Diseases (ICD) mental health chapter until 2019 (WHO, 2020). At this time the diagnostic category was redefined as 'gender incongruence', and is now situated within the 'Conditions related to Sexual Health' ICD chapter. This placement is interesting insofar as it points to an existing classification structure which doesn't, or perhaps cannot, account for experiences that do not easily fit within existing biomedical category frameworks. Indeed, we can interpret these various moves as insights into the (ongoing) shifting medical discourses that frame transgender people's experiences, and which have (re)framed trans(ition) possibilities.

However, the categorisations of transgender experiences sit alongside a medical health care system that remains difficult to enter into and participate in for people with diverse genders and sexualities. Structures of cisnormativity and heterosexism – ideologies which assume people are both cisgender and heterosexual – are embedded in health infrastructures, leaving people living with diverse genders and sexualities largely invisible across all levels of healthcare systems (Baker & Beagan, 2014; Lombardi, 2001). Gaps in cultural competencies contribute to an unclear or inconsistent understanding of the experiences and needs of these individuals and communities, resulting in a lack of appropriate knowledge regarding transgender healthcare (Carabez, Eliason, & Martinson, 2016). More broadly, as Moon (2011) argues, the experiences of those living with diverse genders and sexualities are often mis-aligned with general practice models of gender/sexuality, and are not included in mainstream healthcare teaching practice. These have substantial impacts for healthcare (Schilt & Lagos, 2017). Pearce, Steinberg, and Moon (2019, p. 6) argue that gaps in clinical education regarding the diversity of needs and experiences among transgender people have 'left practitioners without adequate conceptual models for their work, and [...] patients who do not "fit" on the expected spectra feeling underserved and misunderstood'. We have documented a critical example of the problematic impacts of this in describing the 'inappropriate curiosity' that many transgender people report of healthcare professionals objectifying their transgender patients as opportunities for an educational experience (Shepherd, Hanckel, & Guise, 2019), directly resulting from the limitations of general practice models and knowledge accessible to the healthcare professional.

To understand how these histories and the embedded structures of cisnormativity and heterosexism impact on transgender experiences of healthcare, we turn to Pearce's (2018) work, which distinguishes between discourses of 'trans as condition', and 'trans as movement'. The former posits that 'trans' is conditional in the sense that it is something to be defined by a healthcare professional and through transitioning, being trans becomes resolved and 'resolvable' (Pearce, 2018, p. 9). This (often medical) framing assumes a particular trajectory of transition and binary categorisations of male/female. In this sense, there is a way 'to be' trans, and attempts to exist outside of this preconceived notion are rendered invisible. In comparison, 'trans as movement' suggests that 'trans' cannot be defined in a categoric way and instead alludes to the fluid nature of subjective social experiences (Pearce, 2018). This understanding of 'trans' positions transgender as a social identity rather than a defect that needs correcting, creating the possibility of trans individuals who may not want to transition, or to follow non-linear transition paths. Thus, in this framing, 'being' trans is not a finite experience, and brings visibility to previously invisible states of existences. 'Trans as movement' can also work to trouble the transgender/cisgender binary, opening up space for thinking about trans lives through what Latham (2016; 2019) has argued is a multiplicity that takes into account the 'complex ways of being trans' (Latham, 2016, p. 349). As Latham poses,

> Rethinking transexuality as multiple, rather than singular, provides us the opportunity to rethink – and reconstitute – trans medicine. How might we know (and do) transexuality differently? How might more trans ontologies be made possible? (Latham, 2019, p. 15)

Taking up Latham's (2019) proposal to (re)think trans in terms of multiplicity, we consider how the processes and experiences of transitioning for transgender adults are represented in written documents used by the National Health Service (NHS) in England for their care provision, against a backdrop of trans peoples' lived experiences of receiving this care.

Methods

This study employed a mixed-methods approach, including in-depth interviews with trans people, and an analysis of NHS documents used in trans care guidance. We sought to investigate how lived experiences of transitioning align or misalign with care provision advice, and the ontologies of transition embedded within this guidance.

Document analysis

A document analysis was conducted on publicly accessible documents used to guide those practicing within the domain of NHS England in their care provision for transgender adults (aged 18 years or above). Whilst acknowledging that regional and local policies/guidelines may differ, our aim was to compare national level guidance and advice regarding the process of transitioning on which healthcare workers are expected to base their clinical practice decisions. The remit of the search comprised websites operated by NHS England, their regulators and subcontracted bodies, as well as websites operated by organisations representing staff employed by the NHS. Search terms used for identifying documents were: transgender; transition; transition*; trans; trans*; gender identity clinic; gender identity; gender identity service; gender affirming care; gender confirming care; gender dysphoria; nonbinary; non-binary; non binary.

The search was limited to online documents written in English and created in England. As such, the language of transgender health used in the findings reflects the terminology conventionally used in England. The search was conducted between February and April 2020, and included current and past documents providing national level guidance and advice on the process of transitioning. No date limit was used as we wanted to monitor change over time – a key strength of undertaking a document analysis (Bowen, 2009; Wesley, 2014). Whilst a limitation of this approach is that older documents may no longer be retrievable (Bowen, 2009; Wesley, 2014), our goal was to identify narratives of trans(ition) that emerged in publicly accessible documents. The documents included training curricula, service specifications, and care guidelines; see Document References for a full list. Documents were not included if they solely related to transgender youth under the age of 18; did not relate to the process of transitioning; were not related to clinical practice; or did not concern national level advice, such as local prescribing guidelines or equality policies. The quality of documents was assessed following Bowen's (2009) guidance; documents were excluded if they did not address any part of the research question.

Documents were analysed in two steps: a content analysis to identify relevant passages and general themes, followed by a thematic analysis to examine patterns within and across documents (Bowen, 2009; Wesley, 2014). The documents were analysed and considered within the context of their production by considering the date, purpose for their creation, and target audience (Bowen, 2009).

In-depth interviews

The interviews were conducted by the first author, a binary trans man, in July 2019. The study had ethics approval by the King's College London BDM Research Ethics Subcommittee (Approval Number: HR-18/19-11408). A purposive sampling methodology was used to recruit a range of experiences (Etikan, 2016). A recruitment flyer was distributed in online trans spaces for trans people in England, including Facebook groups and dedicated forums, inviting interested individuals to contact the first author. Participants were eligible to take part in an interview if they identified as transgender, were registered with a General Practitioner (GP) in England, and were aged 21 or over. There was no requirement for participants to have transitioned either socially or medically. To minimise bias and pressure to participate, knowing the first author in a personal capacity was an exclusion factor (Adams et al., 2017). Participants were offered a £10 gift voucher to compensate them for their time and emotional labour. As Vincent (2018) has argued, researchers demonstrate respect for the trans community by providing monetary compensation for their time and expertise, demonstrating a commitment to using institutional powers to benefit, rather than exploit this community. The interview schedule was piloted with trans people prior to its use. Participants were given at least 24 h before the interview as a cooling off period to consider whether they wanted to participate (Wilson, Draper, & Ives, 2008), and could withdraw their data within 4 weeks of completing the interview.

In total 8 transgender participants took part in a face-to-face ($n = 1$) or Skype ($n = 7$) interview. All participant names are pseudonyms, and demographic information provided about each participant in the findings adopts the language (e.g. female, trans man, non binary) participants used to describe themselves. Participants were located in a range of urban and regional areas in England. Three participants were women, and two were men. Two were non-binary and agender people, and one participant described herself as a 'detransitioned woman'. One of the limitations of this study is the limited diversity of ethnicity in the sample with all participants identifying as white British or another white background.

Findings

The findings presented below discuss the ways the language around trans identities shifted over time in the documents, and the tensions that emerge vis-à-vis the participants' lived experiences of medical transition(s). Our findings show how our respondents navigated the gender liminal space produced through transitioning, and how the (in)visible moments of agency, resistance, as well as struggles, which remain (un)accounted for in medical documents, contrasted with their lived experiences of transition.

Shifting discourses of trans(itioning)

Chronologically, there has been a shift in the discourse employed in England to describe what 'trans' means. In the two 2008 documents, for instance, binary notions of gender were explicitly referred to:

> Everyone has a gender – man or woman. (Department of Health, 2008, p. 8)

> Gender variance [...] describes the personal discomfort experienced by individuals whose psychological identification as men or as women (the gender identity) is inconsistent with their phenotype (GIRES, 2008, p. 4)

Here, a binary discourse of trans delineates what is visible and invisible by suggesting that transition occurs along a linear gender spectrum. Gendered experiences outside of male 'or' female are unimaginable, and efforts to move beyond this binary become indiscernible. This is a stark contrast to later accounts, such as RCN (2016, p. 5), which asserts that 'gender identity is not necessarily fixed and can be fluid over time'.

It is notable that no documents published between 2009 and 2012 were retrievable. As Pearce (2018, p. 70) notes, the restructuring of the NHS in 2012 led to many documents, trans related and others, being permanently archived. However, the available data suggests that there was a shift in language between these periods, towards 'movement' discourses of gender and being trans. For instance, the RCPsych (2013, p. 12) guidelines stated 'there is growing recognition that many people do not regard themselves as conforming to the binary man/woman divide'. GMC (2015a, pp. 56–57) defined 'gender' as 'a man or a woman' but 'transgender' as 'a person whose self-identity does not conform unambiguously to conventional notions of male or female gender'. RCSLT (2017, p. 11) required trainees to 'understand gender as a continuum' whilst RCSLT (2019, p. 11) required trainees have a 'knowledge of gender identity as an internally experienced and personally defined phenomenon'. It is notable that this shift in language occurred alongside a wider societal shift in how trans(ition) is viewed, evidenced in changes to policy.

The two documents from 2008 were written when Gender Reassignment – the protective characteristic for transgender people in U.K. equality legislation – was legally defined in the U.K. as a 'process which is undertaken under medical supervision' (Department of Health, 2008, p. 33), demarcating transition as a 'process' managed and manageable by health professionals. Superseded by the Equality Act 2010, Gender Reassignment then came to be understood more broadly, with NHS England and NHS Improvement (2019, p. 12) indicating: 'it is enough if [a trans person is] undergoing a personal process of changing gender'. This legal shift, alongside increased representations of trans people in popular culture and digital media have afforded increased visibility of trans activists voices, and increased visibility of the trans population more broadly (Hines, 2013; Pearce, 2018). Within the healthcare context, this has contributed to a broader reframing of transitioning. Correspondingly, the most recent service specifications for Gender Identity Clinics (GICs) in England actively promote the provision of individualised transitions: 'Individuals on the gender dysphoria pathway will have different needs, and the pathway will not always be linear or sequential' (NHS England and NHS Improvement, 2019, p. 7). This shift away from a disease-based model toward an identity-based model of trans(ition) reconstructs the entry point(s) into medical transition to enable trans individuals to have greater agency over their bodies as they engage with the medical system, making previously invisible, non-linear transition paths visible. Whilst seemingly progressive, the pre-condition of a diagnosis for accessing medical interventions still demands that an underlying pathology of gender dysphoria be established – the narrative of 'being born in the wrong body', which has been appropriately critiqued as not applying to all trans experiences (Latham, 2019). Although the documents (Barrett, 2017; Department of Health, n.d.; NHS England, 2017b) affirmed that 'transsexualism'/ 'gender dysphoria' was not considered a mental health problem, NHS England (2018, p. 6) indicated that: 'We therefore take the view that the commissioning obligation depends on a clinical diagnosis of gender dysphoria from a specialist clinical team'. Latham (2019, p. 4) has argued this diagnostic pre-requisite works to performatively reproduce 'sex, gender and "gender dysphoria" as static, predetermined and independent of medical encounters', which obscures the complex realities of trans people's lives in medicine.

Meeting milestones? Overcoming (im)possibilities in transition

Whilst we see possibilities emerge for reframing transition in these documents, we also see collisions between the discourses of 'trans as movement' and 'trans as condition' in the interviews. The predetermined milestones that people must reach in order to gain access to individualised medical transitions, as well as the long wait times for accessing GICs (Pitts-Taylor, 2020), can lead to medical transitions being delayed. This was, for instance, the case for Anna (female, aged 31–40) who described the GIC referral process as, 'It's a case of, you get put on this waiting list and then you're almost forgotten about.' Waiting for hormone replacement therapy (HRT) was described as a shared frustration for six participants, five of whom undertook hormone therapy with a private healthcare provider whilst waiting to progress through the NHS GICs. For Rodney (male, aged 31–40), seeking private care was described as a positive experience, in that accessing HRT in a timely manner 'is such a big thing because it should positively impact on my other conditions and, erm, taking testosterone should improve my quality of life'. However, this form of care was not available to others without incurring a substantial personal cost, as Robin indicated:

> Frankly I couldn't afford to get private healthcare anyway, I made some, you know, questionable financial decisions. And, erm, and basically I was thinking about just doing DIY [self-medicating] if I couldn't get private healthcare. (Robin – nonbinary, 21–30 years)

Robin expressed not just a need to start hormones, but a desperation to access the care that they require, going so far as putting themselves at financial risk, and potential harm from pursuing access to hormones without medical oversight. As the provider of universal healthcare in England, the NHS makes health care available free at the point of delivery. Seeking care outside of the NHS is anomalous and the choice to pay privately often needs to be rationalised (and resourced) by individuals (Exley, Rousseau, Donaldson, & Steele, 2012; Gimlin, 2007), a point made by Robin who could not ordinarily afford private healthcare.

Accessing the care one needs is thus not just limited to one's ability to meet the defined conditions outlined above. Some 'milestones' can be (re)negotiated with access to certain forms of capital, particularly economic and (sub)cultural capital/knowledge (Hanckel & Morris, 2014), to source the know-how to seek care elsewhere. This was the case for Hannah, who drew on the sub-cultural knowledge assembled by her local trans community when seeking a GP who she hoped would be more receptive to working with private providers to prescribe HRT:

> And I had a different GP who was known to be good with mental health issues. But actually, I stopped seeing him and started seeing someone else when I started having to do trans healthcare things because I heard from a friend that he wasn't so great with them and trans things. (Hannah – woman, 21–30 years)

Hannah explained that she 'found him on a trans GP list' on the internet. Jack (trans man, aged 41–50) recounted a similar experience finding his GP 'from [the] internet because she was [a] recommended GP on a list of [trans] friendly people'. Whilst each participant invested labour into securing care, some had to invest additional resources to locate local trans communities and resources online. This relied on not only private device access, but also required certain levels of digital literacy and additional labour to navigate digital platforms, including social media, and find information and support online, a point found elsewhere about young trans peoples' engagement across social media platforms (Hanckel, Vivienne, Byron, Robards, & Churchill, 2019). The extra labour that five of our participants had to put in, and the resources they had to invest to locate and access HRT is indicative of a system that does not respond to patient needs. The first author, as a binary trans man with conventional goals for transitioning, has moved through the English GIC system with relative ease. However, he also sought private care to avoid long waiting lists and, as well as being part of trans support groups, this has made him critically conscious of the fact that not everybody has the same transition trajectory or is able to access (aspects of) transition without connections to wider support networks, and resources to access those networks and HRT. It is notable that 7 out of 8 participants were recruited through trans organisations and groups; Pearce (2018) has also discussed the collective effort involved in securing care with the advice and help of support groups. Curating (sub)cultural knowledge in this way can work to empower individuals to be engaged actors in healthcare encounters, but does involve a reliance on peer knowledge sharing. These are instances of what Newman et al. (2020) call 'inclusivity labour', that is, the labour that individuals invest in cultivating the care they require.

Living in liminality: confrontations in movement

Discourses of 'transitioning' stipulate the existence of a liminal space between normative expectations of what it means to be a woman or man. Hannah experienced confrontation outside a medical context arising from the antagonistic awareness by other people of her body:

> [T]he last time I went swimming was I think three months into having taken hormones and started developing breasts and then, you know, I had a really bad experience with that, where like, swimming costumes are, you know, tight and everything is visible so people saw like genitals and breasts and like, it was bad. Erm, so I haven't been since. (Hannah – woman, 21–30 years)

Hannah's body problematised the trans/cis binary for onlookers, which works to 'other' trans people, analogously to the delineation of gender 'deviances' in the early twentieth century which pathologised trans identities through a discourse of 'trans as condition'. Her coping mechanism was to exclude herself from participating in this activity, which perpetuates the conditions in which many trans bodies remain invisible. Jane (aged 21–30), who was in the early stages of exploring their agender identity when interviewed, similarly rendered themself invisible by retaining the gender they were assigned at birth on their medical record. Describing their gender, Jane explained that, 'at the moment I feel like I lean more towards male than female but I think that's also me overcompensating for always being gendered female'. Jane speaks to the fluid nature of identity, reminiscent of a 'trans as movement' framing, yet also clarifies that, 'No, I wouldn't probably [change the gender marker on medical record]. Maybe further on if I – it, it depends on like, transitioning and things like that.' Whilst Jane is living in a gender liminal space, this fluidity of gender is made invisible on their official records. Yet they also open the possibility of visibly discerning this fluidity in the future by adopting a different gender marker.

When joining a new GP practice, Helen (female, aged over 71 years) mediated this boundary-crossing question of when to adopt a female gender marker, indicating 'even though I hadn't had the surgery, erm, just simply describing myself as female and leaving it at that'. Although Helen acknowledged surgery as a milestone in her transition, she did not make the credibility of her gender identity conditional on this. Instead, she used her own sense of agency to legitimise herself as a woman while also recognising the conditions of liminality in which she lives, even if the complexity of the liminality disappears through an inflexible form.

In the interviews, gender markers were not only considered to operate as a delimitation to one's identity, but also as hurdles that had to be negotiated in relation to healthcare infrastructures:

> I wanted to change my name to a male, keep my NHS number and – and that's turned out to be, erm, impossible. I mean initially impossible because [...] if I would change the prefix they would have to generate a new NHS number. What is the point to lose all of my medical data? (Jack – trans man, 41–50 years)

Making changes to a gender marker meant that Jack's prior interactions with the healthcare system were erased, leaving him in a different kind of liminality whereby his health is rendered invisible. It is important to note that the negotiations that take place in determining what gender to include on forms, and the emotional labour involved in making these decisions is rendered invisible. This is in part because 'trans' is seen as conditional and thus resolvable, and trans people are expected to fit neatly into existing health structures.

Where this liminal space surfaced in 19 of the 31 documents was in relation to the need for continuing or subsequent healthcare. For instance, a 'name change may lead, for example, to trans women being offered smear tests, and trans men being offered [prostate] tests. In neither case is this appropriate' (GIRES, 2008, p. 19). Other documents also acknowledged the importance of appropriate ongoing screening for trans people (BASHH, 2019; GMC, 2013; PHE, 2019; RCGP, 2019; RCN, 2016, 2017). These documents suggest that transition can in fact create new medical problems for trans people, who as patients are registered as 'male' or 'female', thus limiting their possibilities for being engaged with appropriate future health interventions. At the same time, the documents try to raise awareness of the people who are living in this liminality. Pregnancy, for example, is normatively understood as unique to women. However, FSRH (2019b, p. 5), as well as FSRH (2017, 2018, 2019a), indicated that, 'Trans-men can have pregnancies and may opt for abortion'. As Toze (2018) notes, the phenomenon of male pregnancy has yet to attain social acceptance. The possibility for trans men and non-binary people to be pregnant thus only becomes conceivable in the medical system when there are imaginable future health impacts linked to this liminal space.

Trans as 'movement' here is medically defined through pre-existing categories employed to monitor and regulate health, raising the concern that some patients will not be provided with the health care they need and deserve. Our participants' actions were regulated through such categorisation and the 'trans as movement' framework surfaces these confrontations. We argue that a 'trans as movement' framing might also shift the liminal space from a moment between normative expectations, and make possible a more expansive ontology of gender, to account for multiplicities of tran(sition) trajectories. This conceptual tool could have substantive implications for healthcare systems, as well as for trans people, like Hannah, where it could be used to dislocate the ontological violence that the gender binary performs. For Hannah then this might mean she positions her body at the swimming pool as neither pathological nor between a binary, but rather as a simple, unproblematic element of a multiplicity of trajectories of trans(ition).

Moving beyond transition: limitless frontiers?

Across the documents, transitioning was most commonly conceptualised as a 'process of change from the gender role associated with sex assigned at birth to another gender role' (RCPsych, 2018, p. 6). Various outcome measures for this were noted, such as 'achieving personal authenticity' (GIRES, 2008, p. 39) or positing that medical intervention 'ends when the patient is happy and functioning confidently in their acquired [male or female] gender role' (Department of Health, 2008, p. 87). Such imagined endings infer that transitioning is a limited process where people move to(ward) their desired gender, with transition being realised when they have arrived at it. Clune-Taylor (2019), in their study of the management of intersex conditions, argue that treatment is directed towards 'cisgendered futures', which has resonances with the medical treatment inferred to in the medical guidance documents pertaining to trans bodies. Through the narrow rendering of trans identities in medical contexts, medical interventions become aligned with a linear trajectory of treatment to clinically produce 'cisgendered lives'.

These nominal closures frame transitioning both as movement, and as conditional, in that 'movement' is made possible but always contained within a health framework of 'condition'. However, an alternative view of transition as limitless also surfaced in the documents, for example:

> Although gender variance is alleviated to a greater or lesser extent by treatment, to the point that many individuals say that they no longer experience any discomfort, they may, nonetheless, continue to need hormone therapy and monitoring throughout life. (GIRES, 2008, p. 5)

The indefiniteness of taking HRT from a medical perspective suggests that transition is, debatably, never concluded. For example, Helen and Hannah discussed the role that HRT played in their lives:

> So you just kind of get used to [new medication] in the same way that I get used to slapping a [hormone] patch on every five days [...] . (Helen – female, aged 71 years or over)

> In terms of what my GP has to deal with, like I've done all the things already. Like you know there is no more referrals coming through, so they just have to hand over my prescription and read the letters from [the GIC], so things are pretty settled. (Hannah – woman, 21–30 years)

Whilst both of these participants have, in a sense, culminated their transitions in that there is no additional medical intervention planned, they will nonetheless continue to have lifelong interactions with the healthcare system in continuing to access gender-affirming hormones.

Alex: a vignette

We conclude this section with Alex's experience, which talks to the complexity of the liminal space and intersection of 'trans as condition' and 'trans as movement' in an individual's life. During recruitment, Alex (aged 21–30) described herself as being a 'detransitioned woman', having previously identified as a trans man in the early 2010s. As we discuss below, Alex uses the restrictive language of 'detransition' to articulate her nebulous position of being neither simply cis nor trans. When asked to explain how she currently understands her gender identity, she said that:

> I describe myself as female because I am, and that is a fact that I cannot escape from. I describe myself as a trans person because I did [medically] transition for many years and that is also a fact. Beyond that I don't get into words about feelings because it's more undetermined – if I started I would never stop.

Around the time Alex medically transitioned, the documents we analysed privileged an understanding of transitioning which was oriented towards 'trans as condition', offering limited movement in how someone transitions, and the presumed linearity of this experience. Alex observed this linear progression, but found it to conflict with her lived experience:

> I found that [transitioning] re-focused how I felt about my body in different ways and that I was not less dysphoric, I was dysphoric about different things in different ways.

Detransitioning is conventionally conceptualised as unfixing transition, as Alex noted when discussing other people's reactions:

> People are like, 'Oh so you're going back to being a nice, normal lady and wearing pink dresses', and it's like, no. Like, I'm like this. If you say that you're like, if you describe what you're doing, and oh I'm not taking testosterone anymore, then that goes down a lot better. But the flip side is you lose the specificness of what you're doing.

A misalignment of perspectives on what detransitioning means is presented here. Alex's use of the term 'detransition' should not to be seen to represent the reversal of a linear model of transition, that is, a movement back to one's previous self. Rather, detransition for Alex is described as a forward-oriented movement, experienced as a process of gaining a deeper understanding of herself. What is interesting here is the way that Alex employed the concept of detransition to claim space for her own experience in a context in which transition has been medicalised. The use of this term appears to support the work of de-medicalising her body, as part of a movement away from medical transition(s). She acknowledged that describing her experience in medical terms, such as 'not taking testosterone anymore', enabled her to be more easily understood, yet this erased the complexity of her movement to(ward) a more fluid, open-ended future that acknowledges the multiplicity and shape-shifting character of gender, which current medical discourse cannot offer and/or make possible.

Discussion

This paper has shown how the complexity of transition(s) is depicted but also obscured in documents used by NHS England in their care provision for transgender adults. Examining our participants' lived experiences of medical transition alongside healthcare guidance, we have examined the shifting field of healthcare provision that has (attempted) to accommodate gender diverse experiences, drawing on Pearce's (2018) framework of 'trans as movement' and 'trans as condition'. This work has surfaced existing gaps and tensions in an identity-based model of transition operating within the constraints of a biomedical healthcare system, as well as demonstrating what becomes (in)visible in the gender liminal space that medical transitions necessitate. Extending Pearce's work, we have shown that some specific ontologies of transition were revealed through the analysis, which had changed over time through the documents. These ontologies of transitioning, as we have shown, could not account for all lived experiences, especially gender fluidity.

Our findings point to the complex and creative ways in which transgender people are responding to often restrictive ontologies of medical transition. It is notable that transgender people often have to do additional, deliberate work to fit themselves into the pre-existing options for categorisation, evidenced by our participants' attempts to negotiate gender liminal space in medical forms. Furthermore, we also see how our participants' access to healthcare had to be renegotiated at critical moments where they faced confrontations with wait times, for example, and had to locate their experience in relation to the imposition of predetermined medical milestones. What remains invisible are the many ways in which transgender people navigate these confrontations with health guidelines that are mis-aligned with experience, and how this becomes regulated for those who do not have access to the economic capital and associated (sub)cultural capital required to navigate these structures beyond, but always in relation to, the healthcare provider.

In the documents, an understanding of transition as moving to an alternative gender role was identified. This presupposes that there is an end point to transitioning. Deutsch et al. (2013) have discussed the requirements for medical records to be inclusive of trans people so that they do not seek to conclude a transition. Our analysis extends this argument, pointing to the need for medical records to capture the complexity of ongoing transition(s) and recognise the labour involved in negotiating these processes; labour that extends well beyond existing fixed biomedical discourses. Bauer et al. (2009) have described the systemic cisnormativity that perpetuates the institutional erasure of trans people, in part through administrative procedures. We argue that this also works to maintain trans/cis binaries and a discourse of 'trans as condition' by imagining the '*fixed*', '*fixable*' and/or '*resolvable*' moments at an (imagined) ending (Pearce, 2018, p. 9). Trans people, we argue, move toward an alternative, which is not to say that an identity becomes 'resolvable', but rather that this continuous movement speaks to the fluid and entangled nature of living with transition(s) and gender possibilities, as exemplified by Alex's experience of detransitioning. Whilst acknowledging the possible spatial and temporal contexts that regulate a 'trans as movement' framing, we are also optimistic about the (as yet unrealised) possibilities of this framework, and the work that it can do in confronting the ontological violence that the gender binary performs.

Pearce's (2018) work attests to the movement that many people go through as they transition away from their assigned gender at birth. Our interviewees demonstrated how this movement is ongoing and may lead to further reconfiguration(s) of the self at a future point in time. Sociologists have long spoken about the ongoing work on the self (Giddens, 1991). However, the structures of biomedical discourse located in specific socio-historical contexts have directed the (im)possibilities of ontologies of trans(ition), which have restricted this ongoing process of work on the self for transgender people as one that occurs only within healthcare contexts, and regulated by and towards biomedical imagined 'cisgender futures'. Future studies in medical sociology could focus on interrogating the (im)possible healthcare trajectories that we have identified in healthcare guidance and practice, and undertake studies that attend to the variety of ways in which structural norms (i.e. gender) become embedded in the discourses and practices of healthcare and the imagined futures of those who receive medical intervention(s). In addition, there is much sociological work that this analysis suggests is required in challenging the temporalities assumed within the design of trans health systems, which currently restrict many transgender people to a representation of their health care needs as linear, medically-oriented, and consistently stable over time.

Concluding comments

As we have shown, advocating for widening the possibilities through which trans people and trans bodies come into existence and are recognised in the medical field is insufficient if this advocacy does not take account of the very real lived experiences of these people. As a conceptual tool, 'trans as movement' can be used to create space for more expansive ontologies of gender that confront the harms and restrictions imposed by the gender binary, and offer alternative ways of (re)imagining multiplicity in trans(ition) trajectories and futures for both those in healthcare delivery, and for trans patients. Advocates could mobilise this framework as a tool for rethinking care articulations in health policies, guidelines and training curricula for emerging health professionals to enable individualised needs to be realised and responded to. Future studies in this area should also highlight the additional intersectional experiences of transgender people, which must inform and contribute to future healthcare guidance whilst ensuring that the multiplicity of transgender lives are understood to ensure supportive and relevant guidance is provided as it relates to transition. To this end, interventions which not only enhance trans people's experiences of healthcare, but also recognise the limitations of current practices, are imperative to furthering conceptualisations of trans(ition) which can better account for those whose existences are, as of now, unimaginable and indiscernible.

Acknowledgements

We would like to thank our participants for their time and emotional labour in speaking with us and sharing their experiences.

Disclosure statement

No potential conflict of interest was reported by the author(s).

References

Adams, N., Pearce, R., Veale, J., Radix, A., Castro, D., Sarkar, A., & Thom, K. C. (2017). Guidance and ethical considerations for undertaking transgender health research and institutional review boards adjudicating this research. *Transgender Health, 2*, 165–175.

Baker, K., & Beagan, B. (2014). Making assumptions, making space: An anthropological critique of cultural competency and its relevance to queer patients. *Medical Anthropology Quarterly, 28*(4), 578–598.

Bauer, G. R., Hammond, R., Travers, R., Kaay, M., Hohenadel, K. M., & Boyce, M. (2009). 'I don't think this is theoretical; this is our lives': How erasure impacts health care for transgender people. *Journal of the Association of Nurses in AIDS Care, 20*, 348–361.

Bowen, G. (2009). Document analysis as a qualitative research method. *Qualitative Research Journal, 9*(2), 27–40.

Carabez, R. M., Eliason, M. J., & Martinson, M. (2016). Nurses' knowledge about transgender patient care. *ANS. Advances in Nursing Science, 39*(3), 257–271.

Clune-Taylor, C. (2019). Securing cisgendered futures: Intersex management under the 'disorders of sex development' treatment model. *Hypatia, 34*, 690–712.

Davy, Z., & Toze, M. (2018). What is gender dysphoria? A critical systematic narrative review. *Transgender Health, 3*(1), 159–169.

Deutsch, M. B., Green, J., Keatley, J., Mayer, G., Hastings, J., Hall, A. M., ... Blumer, O. (2013). Electronic medical records and the transgender patient: Recommendations from the world professional association for transgender health EMR working group. *Journal of the American Medical Informatics Association, 20*(4), 700–703.

Drescher, J. (2010). Queer diagnoses: Parallels and contrasts in the history of homosexuality, gender variance, and the diagnostic and statistical manual. *Archives of Sexual Behavior, 39*, 427–460.

Etikan, I. (2016). Comparison of convenience sampling and purposive sampling. *American Journal of Theoretical and Applied Statistics, 5*, 1.

Exley, C., Rousseau, N., Donaldson, C., & Steele, J. G. (2012). Beyond price: Individuals' accounts of deciding to pay for private healthcare treatment in the UK. *BMC Health Services Research, 12*, 53.

Foucault, M. (1978). *The will to knowledge. The history of sexuality. Volume 1: An introduction.* (R. Hurley, Trans.). New York, NY: Vintage Books.

Giddens, A. (1991). *Modernity and self-identity* (1st ed.). Stanford, CA: Stanford University Press.

Gimlin, D. (2007). Accounting for cosmetic surgery in the USA and Great Britain: A cross-cultural analysis of women' narratives. *Body & Society*, *13*(1), 41–60.

Hanckel, B., & Morris, A. (2014). Finding community and contesting heteronormativity: Queer young people's engagement in an Australian online community. *Journal of Youth Studies*, *17* (7), 872–886.

Hanckel, B., Vivienne, S., Byron, P., Robards, B., & Churchill, B. (2019). 'That's not necessarily for them': LGBTIQ+ young people, social media platform affordances and identity curation. *Media, Culture & Society*, *41*, 1261–1278.

Hines, S. (2013). *Gender diversity, recognition and citizenship: Towards a politics of difference*. London: Springer.

Latham, J. R. (2016). Trans men' sexual narrative-practices: Introducing STS to trans and sexuality studies. *Sexualities*, *19*(3).

Latham, J. R. (2019). Axiomatic: Constituting 'transexuality' and trans sexualities in medicine. *Sexualities*, *22*, 1–2, 347–368.

Law, J., & Benschop, R. (1997). Resisting pictures: Representation, distribution and ontological politics. *The Sociological Review*, *45*(S1), 158–182.

Lev, A. I. (2013). Gender dysphoria: Two steps forward, one step back. *Clinical Social Work Journal*, *41*, 288–296.

Lombardi, E. (2001). Enhancing transgender health care. *American Journal of Public Health*, *91*(6), 869–872.

Moon, L. (2011). The gentle violence of therapists: Misrecognition and dis-location of the other. *Psychotherapy and Politics International*, *9*(3), 194–205.

Newman, C. E., Prankumar, S. K., Cover, R., Rasmussen, M. L., Marshall, D., & Aggleton, P. (2020). Inclusive health care for LGBTQ+ youth: Support, belonging, and inclusivity labour. *Critical Public Health*, 1–10.

Pearce, R. (2018). *Understanding trans health*. Bristol: Policy Press.

Pearce, R., Steinberg, D. L., & Moon, I. (2019). Introduction: The emergence of 'trans'. *Sexualities*, *22*(1–2), 3–12.

Pitts-Taylor, V. (2020). 'A slow and unrewarding and miserable pause in your life': Waiting in medicalized gender transition. *Health*, *24*(6), 646–664.

Rubin, H. (1999). Trans studies: Between a metaphysics of presence and absence. In K. More & S. Whittle (Eds.), *Reclaiming genders: Transsexual grammars at the Fin de Siècle* (pp. 173–192). New York, NY: Cassell.

Schilt, K., & Lagos, D. (2017). The development of transgender studies in sociology. *Annual Review of Sociology*, *43*(1), 425–443.

Shepherd, A., Hanckel, B., & Guise, A. (2019). Trans health and the risks of inappropriate curiosity. *BMJ Opinion*. Retrieved from https://blogs.bmj.com/bmj/2019/09/09/trans-health-and-the-risks-of-inappropriate-curiosity/

Sumerau, J. (2020). Expanding transgender studies in sociology. *Sociological Inquiry*, *90*, 217–225.

Toze, M. (2018). The risky womb and the unthinkability of the pregnant man: Addressing trans masculine hysterectomy. *Feminism & Psychology*, *28*(2), 194–211.

Toze, M. (2020). Specialization and minority health care: Hormone therapy for trans people in England. *Journal of Health Services Research & Policy*, *25*(4), 246–251.

Vincent, B. (2018). Studying trans: Recommendations for ethical recruitment and collaboration with transgender participants in academic research. *Psychology & Sexuality*, *9*(2), 102–116.

Wesley, J. (2014). The qualitative analysis of political documents. In Bertie Kaal, Isa Maks, & Annemarie van Elfrinkhof (Eds.), *From text to political positions: Text analysis across disciplines, discourse approaches to politics, society and culture* (pp. 135–160). Amsterdam: John Benjamins Publishing Company.

WHO. (2020). WHO/Europe brief – transgender health in the context of ICD-11. Euro.who.int. Retrieved from http://www.euro.who.int/en/health-topics/health-determinants/gender/gender-definitions/whoeurope-brief-transgender-health-in-the-context-of-icd-11

Wilson, S., Draper, H., & Ives, J. (2008). Ethical issues regarding recruitment to research studies within the primary care consultation. *Family Practice*, *25*, 456–461.

Document References

Barrett, J. (2017). Gender dysphoria: Assessment and management for non-specialists. *BMJ*, *357*, j2866.

BASHH. (2019). BASHH recommendations for integrated sexual health services for trans, including non-binary, people [PDF file]. Retrieved from https://bit.ly/2H3en6a

Department of Health. (2008). Trans: A practical guide for the NHS [PDF file]. Retrieved from https://bit.ly/3pxWZIg

Department of Health. (n.d.). Gender dysphoria services: A guide for general practitioners and other healthcare staff [PDF file]. Retrieved from https://bit.ly/32NoIL7

FSRH. (2018). FSRH consultation response: Consultation on a new version of the GP Curriculum by the Royal College of General Practitioners [PDF file]. Retrieved from https://bit.ly/38QjvWP

FSRH. (2019a). Advanced Clinical Practitioner (ACP) integrated sexual health and HIV specialist training curriculum [PDF file]. Retrieved from https://bit.ly/3nqn2PK

FSRH. (2019b). Termination of pregnancy – consultation on draft guideline [PDF file]. Retrieved from https://bit.ly/2K4JTSs

FSRH CEU. (2017). FSRH CEU statement: Contraceptive choices and sexual health for transgender and non-binary people [PDF file]. Retrieved from https://bit.ly/3nkSoY2

GIRES. (2008). Guidance for GPs and other clinicians on the treatment of gender variant people [PDF file]. Retrieved from https://bit.ly/38NFcXp

GMC. (2013). Fitness to practice allegations handbook [PDF file]. Retrieved from https://bit.ly/2UsY6uz

GMC. (2015a). Approving changes to curricula, examinations and assessments: Equality and diversity requirements [PDF file]. Retrieved from https://bit.ly/3lB6rIx

GMC. (2015b). Guidance for colleges on equality and diversity considerations for curricula and assessment system changes draft [PDF file]. Retrieved from https://bit.ly/3nxlBPD

HFEA. (n.d.). Information for trans and non-binary people seeking fertility treatment [PDF file]. Retrieved from https://bit.ly/35zBIG3

NHS England. (2013). Interim gender dysphoria protocol and service guideline [PDF file]. Retrieved from https://bit.ly/36Hi1LJ

NHS England. (2016). Primary care responsibilities in prescribing and monitoring hormone therapy for transgender and non-binary adults (updated) [PDF file]. https://bit.ly/35zzTZV

NHS England. (2017a). Gender identity services for adults (non-surgical interventions) [PDF file]. Retrieved from https://bit.ly/2IDYm7e

NHS England. (2017b). Gender identity services for adults (surgical interventions) [PDF file]. Retrieved from https://bit.ly/3kC3BBw

NHS England. (2017c). Guide to consultation: Specialised gender identity services for adults [PDF file]. Retrieved from https://bit.ly/38SfzVL

NHS England. (2018). Specialised gender identity services for adults; report on outcome of public consultation and update to equality impact assessment [PDF file]. Retrieved from https://bit.ly/2IvlF3B

NHS England. (2019b). Gender identity services for adults (non-surgical interventions) [PDF file]. Retrieved from https://bit.ly/3nvjc8a

NHS England. (2019c). Gender identity services for adults (surgical interventions) [PDF file]. Retrieved from https://bit.ly/36I7bFx

NHS England and NHS Improvement. (2019). Delivering same-sex accommodation [PDF file]. Retrieved from https://bit.ly/2IHr0US

NHS England. (n.d.). Clinical commissioning policy: [Gender identity services] [PDF file]. Retrieved from https://bit.ly/3nx7d9N

PHE. (2019). Information for trans and non-binary people NHS screening programmes [PDF file]. Retrieved from https://bit.ly/2IFJg1p

RCGP. (2019). The role of the GP in caring for gender-questioning and transgender patients [PDF file]. Retrieved from https://bit.ly/3lz4CvK

RCN. (2016). Fair care for trans patients [PDF file]. Retrieved from https://bit.ly/3nqZQ3R

RCN. (2017). Fair care for trans patients [PDF file]. Retrieved from https://bit.ly/2UsECGi
RCPsych. (2013). Good practice guidelines for the assessment and treatment of adults with gender dysphoria [PDF file]. Retrieved from https://bit.ly/32NSmQA
RCPsych. (2018). Supporting transgender and gender-diverse people [PDF file]. Retrieved from https://bit.ly/35ATZmg
RCSLT. (2017). Trans and gender-diverse voice & communication therapy competency framework [PDF file]. Retrieved from https://bit.ly/2H8jMZS.
RCSLT. (2019). Trans and gender-diverse voice & communication therapy competency framework [PDF file]. Retrieved from https://bit.ly/2H4m4cm

Expanding and improving trans affirming care in Australia: experiences with healthcare professionals among transgender young people and their parents

Clare Bartholomaeus, Damien W. Riggs and Annie Pullen Sansfaçon

ABSTRACT

Access to medical care is significant for many transgender young people and their families, which involves interactions with healthcare professionals. While a trans affirming model is used across Australian paediatric gender clinics, this does not automatically mean that all transgender young people and their parents experience the care they receive as affirming. This article considers the experiences and views of transgender young people (aged 11–17) and their parents in relation to healthcare professionals inside and outside of gender clinics in Australia. Ten qualitative interviews were conducted with parent–child dyads in two Australian states. Key themes relating to healthcare professionals were: differing levels of healthcare professional knowledge and affirmation, quality of service is dependent on individual healthcare professionals, and lack of connected services and referral pathways. The discussion explores specific issues arising from the findings that suggest implications for training for healthcare professionals so as to be better equipped to provide trans affirming clinical care.

Introduction

Increasing numbers of transgender young people are presenting to gender clinics for services in Australia and internationally. As a result, more dedicated gender clinics with multidisciplinary teams are emerging (e.g. Chen et al., 2016; Kaltiala et al., 2020; Telfer, Tollit, & Feldman, 2015). Importantly, such clinics exist in the context of broader healthcare services accessed by transgender young people and their families. Previous research on transgender young people's experiences with healthcare professionals provides evidence for both strengths and limitations in the healthcare sector in terms of providing trans affirming clinical care. Trans affirming clinical care is defined as an approach that treats gender diversity as an aspect of human gender expression, and seeks to validate transgender people's experiences of their gender (Chang, Singh, & dickey, 2018). In terms of strengths, professionals who are supportive, knowledgeable, and, respectful – including by using correct names and pronouns – are experienced as affirming (Corliss, Belzer, Forbes, & Wilson, 2007; Guss et al., 2019; Riggs, Bartholomaeus, & Pullen Sansfaçon, 2020; Strauss et al., 2017). Experiences of such affirming responses have been related to high levels of satisfaction among young people and their families attending paediatric gender clinics (Inwards-Breland et al., 2019; Pullen Sansfaçon et al., 2019; Tollit, Feldman, McKie, & Telfer, 2019). In terms of limitations, research has identified a lack of understanding by healthcare professionals of transgender young people's needs, discrimination, misgendering, and a lack of training about gender diversity (Carlile, 2020; Corliss et al., 2007; Eisenberg, McMorris, Rider, Gower, & Coleman, 2020; Goldenberg et al., 2019; Gridley et al., 2016; Guss et al., 2019; Heard et al., 2018; Strauss et al., 2017; Temple Newhook, Benson, Bridger, Crowther, & Sinnott, 2018). Such lack of understanding on the part of healthcare professionals can lead to transgender young people and their parents foregoing care (Clark, Veale, Greyson, & Saewyc, 2018; Goldenberg et al., 2019).

In this article we consider the experiences of transgender young people and their parents in relation to healthcare professionals both inside and outside of paediatric gender clinics in two states in Australia: Victoria and South Australia. There is currently limited research on experiences of Australian gender clinics for young people (aside from Tollit et al., 2019). In Victoria, the *Royal Children's Hospital* provides a comprehensive dedicated gender clinic. In South Australia, a newly named gender clinic exists at the *Women's and Children's Hospital*, offering services specific to transgender young people. Gender services for young people also currently exist in New South Wales, Queensland, and Western Australia. The analysis presented below aims to contribute to the literature by examining some of the more subtle ways in which clinical care may or may not be trans affirming, both in gender clinics and broader healthcare services. In other words, the focus of this article is on how the practices of individual clinicians may be shaped by individual, institutional, and ideological factors that may impact on how transgender young people and their parents experience the clinical care they receive.

Materials and methods

This article draws on an Australian pilot study focused on the clinical care experiences of transgender young people and their families. This Australian project is an iteration of a Canadian study led by the third author (Pullen Sansfaçon, Medico, Suerich-Gulick, & Temple Newhook, 2020) that has also been conducted in the UK and in Switzerland (Medico et al., 2020). Ethics approval for the Australian pilot study was granted by the Flinders University Social and Behavioural Research Ethics Committee and the research ethics board of the University of Montreal.

Reflexivity statement

We are a team of three cisgender researchers who over the past decade have conducted research, engaged in advocacy, and contributed to the provision of training for healthcare professionals in terms of providing trans affirming care. The first author is an academic who works in the social sciences and education, with a particular focus on research with children and young people about gender. The second author is a psychology academic whose research focuses on the lives of transgender people, and who is a psychotherapist who specialises in working with transgender young people from an affirming approach. The third author is a social work academic whose research focuses on the lives of transgender people, and who is a parent of a transgender young person.

Participants and interviews

Information regarding the study was distributed to groups for parents of transgender and gender diverse children, asking parents to contact the research team if they and their child were interested in participating. Inclusion criteria for participating were: (1) being a parent/transgender child dyad willing to be interviewed together (young people aged between 11 and 17), (2) living in South Australia or Victoria, and (3) having received clinical services in relation to gender (from a gender clinic and/or elsewhere).

Upon contacting the research team, potential parent participants were provided with two information sheets: one for themselves, and one for their child. Both information sheets outlined the focus of the project, what was being requested of participants, and contacts should they need support following participation. Having read the applicable information sheet, parents and young people signed a consent form and parents completed a demographic sheet before scheduling an interview. Based on the preferences and location of participants, eight interviews were conducted in person and two interviews were conducted via Skype. The young people in each dyad were provided with a $25 (Australian dollars) voucher for their time. All interviews were conducted by the first author from May-July 2019. Interviews were transcribed by a professional transcription service and pseudonyms were allocated following transcription.

Young people and their parent(s) were interviewed together due to ethics requirements. Dyadic interviews meant that young people had a supportive adult present during the interview, which may have helped allay some fears about being interviewed by a stranger and also assisted with remembering events. However, having a parent present may also have meant that some young people felt that certain topics could not be broached. From our reading of the interview transcripts, however, and as the findings presented below suggest, young people appeared to speak relatively freely about a variety of topics (including their families), in front of their parents. This occasionally included young people disagreeing with the perspectives of their parents, however such disagreements were not evident in the analysis of specific aspects of the data undertaken for the present article.

Interview questions focused on several key topics: coping and resiliency, experience of coming to the clinic, experiences of puberty blockers and/or hormones (if applicable), fertility preservation, and advice to others. Questions were devised for both young people and parents to ensure all participants could contribute, however, participants were invited to add comments at any time.

Analytic approach

An inductive thematic analysis was undertaken of the data, focusing on mentions of healthcare professionals. Other areas of the interviews, including experiences of the receipt of puberty blockers or hormones, are the focus of another article (Riggs et al., 2020). The analytic process was informed by Braun and Clarke (2006): (1) becoming familiar with the data, (2) generating codes, (3) identifying themes, (4) reviewing themes, (5) refining specifics of the themes, and (6) selecting extracts that best illustrate the themes identified. The first author identified all responses in the interview transcripts which mentioned healthcare professionals. This included specific questions relating to healthcare professionals (e.g. how participants decided to see a professional about their gender, their experiences with professionals) and all other mentions of healthcare professionals in the transcripts. Having collated the data set, the first author then read these data extracts repeatedly, developing codes across the set. These broad codes were used to develop specific themes. These themes were confirmed by the second and third authors. Indicative extracts from the interviews were selected to illustrate the themes in the analysis below.

Results

Participant demographics

Ten interviews were conducted in total (five with participants in South Australia and five with participants in Victoria). A total of 21 people participated, as one young person was interviewed with two parents. The average age of the young people participating was 14.3 years (ranging from 11 to 17 years). Of the young people participating, five reported their gender as male, four as female, and one as male and female or non-binary. In terms of current medical care, four young people were in receipt of puberty blockers, two were in receipt of both puberty blockers and hormones, two were in receipt of hormones, and two were not accessing either. The average age of parent participants was 47.3 years (ranging from 38 to 53 years). Of the parent participants, nine reported their gender as female, one as male, and one as non-binary. Of the parent participants, eight reported that they were married or partnered, and three reported that they were divorced or separated. A wide diversity of household yearly income was reported by participants, ranging from under $40,000 to over $150,000 (Australian dollars). Participants were primarily white.

Differing levels of healthcare professional knowledge and affirmation

Trans healthcare guidelines advise that healthcare professionals working with transgender young people should be both affirming and knowledgeable (Oliphant et al., 2018; Telfer, Tollit, Pace, & Pang, 2017; World Professional Association for Transgender Health, 2011). For our participants, however, this was not always the case. Differing experiences of professional knowledge and affirmation are reflected in three subthemes: (1) professionals who were affirming and knowledgeable, (2) professionals who were affirming but lacked knowledge, and (3) professionals who were knowledgeable in their area but were not necessarily affirming.

Professionals who were affirming and knowledgeable

Several of the participants had experiences with healthcare professionals who were both affirming and knowledgeable, and this was most likely to be the case when attending a paediatric gender clinic. For example, Mariah discussed her experiences with a paediatrician and a psychiatrist at a gender clinic:

> They were very positive experiences. They were very professional. I knew that they wanted to help me as quick as possible because the clock was ticking. And they wanted me to feel good, happy, and like my true self. (Mariah, age 17)

Here Mariah indicates that the professionals she engaged with were mindful that delaying treatment can have negative impacts, and that timely access is necessary to ensure the best outcome (Tollit et al., 2019). Similarly, Robyn highlighted her family's positive experiences during their first appointments with a gender clinic:

> It was exciting just to be able to openly discuss it with somebody who knew what they were talking about and to be able to openly express our fears as parents and touch on all those questions that had been building for that amount of time. So, it was a breath for us all, a chance to exhale. (Robyn, parent of Nate, age 16)

Parents may often bring with them fears, as Robyn notes. Professionals who adopt an affirming approach can both listen to such fears, and address them by helping to explore the beliefs that may underpin them.

Professionals who were affirming but lacked knowledge

While it is ideal that healthcare professionals working with transgender young people are both knowledgeable and affirming, professionals may be affirming even when they have not undertaken specific training about working with transgender young people. This was particularly mentioned by participants in terms of general practitioners (GPs). For example, Amanda had seen a GP for treatment for an injury and thought he may be a good GP for her daughter:

Amanda:	I actually made an appointment and went back and explained the situation about Ashleigh and said 'could you be her doctor?' And he said 'yes of course'
Interviewer:	So was he experienced in seeing trans people or …
Amanda:	No. What I found is that even people who aren't experienced, if they're open to listening and learning, we found that doesn't matter. (parent of Ashleigh, age 15)

We suggest, based on the extract from Amanda, that a willingness to be open is a hallmark of a general approach to professional practice that is mindful of the effects of marginalisation upon individuals.

Kya's mother Johannah also highlighted her family's positive experiences with their GP, which Johannah related to the GP's willingness to learn: 'our GP, we were pretty lucky with her, she didn't know a lot but she's learned with us' (Johannah, parent of Kya, age 17). As others have also found with GPs, transgender young people value open-minded professionals who seek to be helpful and understanding, even if they are inexperienced in the area (Strauss et al., 2017).

Professionals who were knowledgeable in their area but not necessarily affirming

In our interviews, it was evident that the professionals seen by participants were very knowledgeable in their profession, yet not necessarily knowledgeable or affirming in terms of working with transgender young people specifically. For example, Miles and Jules discussed a psychologist who Miles saw outside of the gender clinic, whom they both viewed as a good psychologist generally, but who did not seem to have knowledge on working with transgender young people:

> She was good, but I felt like I was educating her on it which wasn't really my job. She was supposed to be helping me. I wasn't supposed to be helping her, really. [...] I think she was a good psychologist and she knew what she was doing. But at the same time, I don't think she was really educated enough on terms and stuff like that. (Miles, age 13)

This experience of needing to educate healthcare professionals is one that has been well documented in relation to both transgender adults (e.g. Riggs, Coleman, & Due, 2014) and transgender young people (e.g. Strauss et al., 2017).

Other participants also noted the difficult balance between being knowledgeable in the general healthcare area and being affirming, including in relation to healthcare professionals they had been referred to for different services outside of paediatric gender clinics:

> The guy at [fertility clinic], he was very informed in his area but not very informed, clearly, in the area of gender diverse people. So, if you're going to be seeing a gender diverse person, if you're in fact the person that they're being referred to, then be informed about them. And know that they're not there to see you because you're necessarily their priority. The fertility is not necessarily their priority; it's just part of their process. (Liz, parent of Jasmine, age 13)

In this extract, Liz is clear that the fertility specialist was well informed about the topic of fertility, yet appeared to have less than adequate knowledge about gender diversity (as has also been found in other studies about fertility preservation, e.g. Bartholomaeus & Riggs, 2020). As Liz notes, the impetus is on healthcare professionals to have adequate knowledge when accepting referrals.

Quality of service is dependent on individual healthcare professionals

From the interviews it was clear that the quality of many services, including at gender clinics, were dependent on the aptitude and commitment of individual healthcare professionals. Reliance upon the trans affirming knowledge of specific professionals may suggest that, at least to some extent, transgender health is seen as solely the province of specialists, rather than being part of general healthcare. This was evident in two sub-themes: (1) significant variation between services provided by different professionals, and (2) reliance on the goodwill and dedication of individual professionals.

Significant variation between professionals

Participants reported significant variation in their experience of different professionals, even within the same service or the same profession. In terms of gender clinics, participants noted that they experienced differing quality of service when engaging with different professionals in the same role. In some cases, it appeared that families were reliant on the care that individual professionals were comfortable providing, and services were provided at their discretion. For example, Liz discussed her family's experiences of a paediatric endocrinologist who was ready to prescribe puberty blockers when they were needed, in contrast to a paediatrician who was less forthcoming:

> They wanted us seeing someone working in what was to become the Gender Clinic. Then we found [paediatrician] completely different. So while [paediatric endocrinologist] was ready to give [blockers] and as soon as it was needed, [paediatrician] had all this red tape, and many papers to read through and sign. A completely different process, which made me realise it wasn't a legal thing, it wasn't even a hospital thing. *It was a doctor-specific requirement.* (emphasis added) (Liz, parent of Jasmine, age 13)

The widest variations in approaches discussed by participants related to GPs and psychologists/counsellors, which may be at least in part attributed to the frequency with which these professionals are sought out by transgender young people and their family outside of gender clinics. For example, Tara highlighted that the first GP they saw had little awareness of other services, whereas the second GP had experience and knowledge:

> the second GP that we saw, but they're at another clinic and they're really hard to get to, he was up on it. He'd had two previous [transgender] children because he focused more on children so he knew exactly, whereas the [first] GP that we saw, they were lovely but no idea who to contact, what sort of support services were out there, anything like that. (Tara, parent of Paul, age 13)

These findings are similar to what Gridley et al. (2016) refer to as 'uncoordinated care', where there are not clear care pathways, and where families may be told by one professional they cannot receive hormones, while another professional is willing to provide them.

Goodwill and dedication of individual professionals

Participants also pointed out very positive experiences with particular healthcare professionals, noting their goodwill and dedication. Notably, across the interviews, two professionals working at gender clinics were frequently referred to as going out of their way to be supportive. For example, Marc highlighted the important role a particular paediatrician had played in their lives:

> she's quite a busy person. She sees so many people and she makes the time to have these one on one conversations and show support. Even when she's not even scheduled to work… she's actually emailed us and done scripts and all sorts of things. She's really there for Mariah in every way. (Marc, parent of Mariah, age 17)

It would seem that this particular professional has adopted a deliberately trans affirming approach that involves going out of one's way to provide support. Other participants discussed how much they liked a particular endocrine nurse who gave puberty blocker injections, including her dedication to the role and the young people she saw:

> the endocrine nurse that gives the injections, I think she just kind of put her hand up and said 'oh, I've given Lupron injections [puberty blockers] before' because some other kids have them for precocious puberty, so she had said 'oh, I can do that.' […] So that was kind of her goodwill, it's not anything official, you know, it's someone just saying 'oh, I can do that injection and I've got space for three kids.' […] But I mean, I always think what happens if she gets really sick or she feels like she might like a new job? (Amanda, parent of Ashleigh, age 15)

While it is clear that these professionals provided important services to participants, it is potentially problematic that services rely on the goodwill and dedication of a small number of professionals.

Lack of connected services and referral pathways

As explored in this third theme, participants noted a lack of connected services and referral pathways, which had the potential to impact on their wellbeing. A lack of connected services, where transgender healthcare is treated as an isolated matter, can mean that transgender health is seen solely as a specialist concern, as we suggested in the previous theme. This was evident in two sub-themes: (1) holistic care and complex needs were not addressed sufficiently at gender clinics, and (2) there was a difficulty in finding additional services needed outside of the gender clinic.

Holistic care and complex needs not addressed sufficiently at gender clinics

Participants discussed needing to seek care outside of gender clinics for two key reasons: additional, more frequent counselling needed for holistic care, and complex needs not being addressed at gender clinics. This, we argue, speaks to broader issues associated with the fact that paediatric clinics consistently face a lack of funding.

Parent participants specifically spoke of the need for further counselling required for their child, for themselves, or for their family as a group. This level of counselling was not available at gender clinics as it was required more frequently and about a broader range of issues:

> we realised that' Jasmine needed a bit more in the way of counselling I suppose, and just individual guidance, which the hospital process doesn't really allow for. If you want to go and chat to someone every few weeks about what's going on, they just don't really have the scope for that, so that's where [psychotherapist] came in. (Liz, parent of Jasmine, age 13)

> it would be lovely if we could have [gender clinic psychologist] locally and see her once or twice a week but we can't do that and really when he's in there all they're really doing is checking in that everything's going okay with gender. They can't help with what most kids really need which is anxiety management and all of that stuff and that's what we really need, I think. (Claudia, parent of Thomas, age 11)

Some of the parent participants discussed the difficulties they had faced in finding services which addressed their children's complex needs. For example, Hunter's child was on the autism spectrum, and found it difficult to find professionals who had experience in both gender and autism:

> I hunted around and went through all the different mental health services, trying to chase up another psychiatrist who could do the assessment who had the experience in both autism and gender, which was a tricky one. We ended up having our first assessment with a guy who was absolutely damaging and jaded, like a court-ordered assessment. (Hunter, parent of Mitch, age 15)

Due to the lack of available services within a gender clinic, Hunter and Mitch were forced to negotiate with a psychiatrist whose views impacted negatively on them.

The difficulty finding affirming services

Finding informed and affirming healthcare professionals could often be difficult for participants. Parent participants discussed their need to be proactive in finding services, and the significant 'trial and error' required before finding the right services. This often occurred prior to receiving services from a gender clinic, given the often long wait times to access gender clinics. For example, Liz noted that she had to proactively look for services in ways which likely would not occur if her child had needed medical services for something else:

> I was given some information to start off with, but I had to proactively pursue a lot of things myself. I called people. I got referrals. I looked into things. It wasn't given to me along the way as just part of the process. I keep going back to a child with any other type of medical concern gets told, 'We'll refer you to this person, and we'll give you this and we'll give this'. (Liz, parent of Jasmine, age 13)

Amelie also noted that counselling services in particular did not know about other services available and that more awareness of other services was needed:

> I feel like the [counselling services] need to know a lot more about other groups, because I find that a lot of groups and counselling, they only know about the hospital and a couple of other counsellors, and then with supportive groups that just know about themselves. I feel like everyone just needs to know about everyone. (Amelie, age 12)

These views clearly document a need for more connected and integrated services and for effective referrals between affirming healthcare professionals. This has been reflected in other research, where transgender young people and their families found out about other services through 'word of mouth' from their friends and other community members (Corliss et al., 2007). That there is not a more systematic approach to providing affirming transgender healthcare indicates the marginal and precarious position of those who are seeking to secure access to quality care in this domain.

Discussion

This article adds to the existing research by considering interactions with healthcare professionals both inside and outside of gender clinics in order to provide a broader and more complex picture of what healthcare needs and experiences can look like for transgender young people and their parents. Overall, and as expected, transgender young people and their parents received more informed and affirming care from dedicated gender clinics than from broader healthcare services. Largely positive experiences of care in gender clinics reflects the existing limited number of studies with young people and their families in Australia (Tollit et al., 2019), Canada (Pullen Sansfaçon et al., 2019), and the US (Inwards-Breland et al., 2019). Receiving such care is particularly important for those accessing medical treatment (puberty blockers and hormones). However, as the findings suggest, healthcare professionals can act as facilitators or barriers to treatment, including in paediatric gender clinics.

Further in regard to paediatric gender clinics, participants noted that the services they received within clinics varied between professionals – particularly in terms of some professionals being more conservative in their approach – and participants describing feeling grateful for and reliant on the goodwill and dedication of individual professionals. It was also apparent that professionals at gender clinics were not always in a position to provide the frequency and level of services needed (particularly counselling) or to address the full range of complex needs of some young people. Finally, it appeared that gender clinics rarely provided recommendations for affirming and knowledgeable healthcare professionals and services outside the clinics, and it was usually up to parents to seek out the additional services needed. Specifically, we note that, at least in our sample, the work of negotiating referrals and linked up care was primarily the responsibility of mothers, constituting a specific form of emotional labour (see Riggs et al., 2020). While, as we note below, some parents appreciated the support provided by gender clinics, this does not necessarily mitigate the emotional labour involved.

Transgender young people and their parents described a diversity of experiences with healthcare professionals outside of gender clinics. Interactions with GPs can be significant for transgender young people and their parents, particularly early on when seeking services and support (e.g. Strauss et al., 2017). In addition, GPs are often relied upon to provide written referrals to other services, such as gender clinics and psychologists. It was clear that experiences with GPs varied, particularly in terms of levels of affirmation and knowledge. Psychologists and counsellors outside of gender clinics can also be particularly important both initially and when more counselling is needed outside of a paediatric gender clinic. However, experiences with psychologists and counsellors outside of gender clinics were also mixed, and for some resulted in potentially damaging experiences.

Overall, the findings we present in this article provide evidence for a number of opportunities for improvement in the provision of trans affirming healthcare, as well as insights regarding the social and structural factors that shape the provision of and engagement of this form of care. The first of these pertains to the effects of cisgenderism in and on healthcare practice. As defined by Ansara and colleagues, cisgenderism refers to 'the discriminatory ideology that delegitimises people's own designations of their genders and bodies' (Ansara & Hegarty, 2013, p. 162). Cisgenderism can take more overt forms (e.g. pathologising gender diversity, silencing conversations about gender diversity), as well as more subtle forms (e.g. a lack of awareness about gender diversity). When discussing their experiences with dedicated gender clinics, it is unsurprising that it was rare for overt cisgenderism to be mentioned by participants (although, as the findings suggest, overt cisgenderism still occurs outside of paediatric gender clinics). Nonetheless, more subtle forms of cisgenderism were arguably evident, even in the accounts of those who reported satisfaction with their care. This includes examples discussed in which transgender health is seen to be the sole responsibility of specialists and, related to this, when wait lists become greatly extended due to lack of funding, leading to immense distress among those waiting to gain access to the care they need. This suggests a pressing need for continued advocacy about how cisgenderism as an ideology impacts upon the healthcare experiences of transgender young people and their parents in Australia, even in a context in which the model of care is arguably more affirming and accessible than in much of the rest of the world.

Additionally, it is important to recognise that knowledge is still developing in some areas of trans affirming care, and there is not always definitive medical knowledge that healthcare professionals can rely upon (e.g. shuster, 2016). For professionals working outside of gender clinics, supports for their work may be less clear and they may need to seek out resources and training themselves. Training is thus a vital component suggested by the present article in terms of both initial education in the context of universities and other tertiary institutions, and continued professional development. Importantly, training on trans affirming healthcare should be provided to *all* healthcare professionals, not just those who specialise in the area, and needs to take into account the specifics of working with young people and their families. Such training needs to be mindful of the effects of cisgenderism – both its overt and more subtle forms – and actively seek to provide education for healthcare professionals as to how they can seek to avoid enacting and reproducing cisgenderism in clinical care. Blakey and Treharne (2019), for example, advocate for the importance of the inclusion of paid transgender community members in the training of healthcare professionals. Importantly, this is not simply to include the lived experience of transgender people, but also to learn from the specific knowledges that transgender people hold about what constitutes trans affirming care, including in recognising, naming and challenging the effects of cisgenderism. Training in this way of conceptualising it extends beyond a problem of 'awareness', to insist that healthcare institutions have a responsibility and the opportunity to address the many ways in which their systems are designed on cisgenderist assumptions, and must be rethought at every level if they are to become truly trans affirming in their practice. Healthcare professionals of all genders can be impacted by institutional cisgenderism in their workplaces and professions, impacting on the care they are able to provide.

There are a growing number of resources available to professionals. Along with the World Professional Association for Transgender Health's (2011) *Standards of Care*, there are professional guidelines for working with transgender people and their families, such as the *Australian Standards of Care and Treatment Guidelines: For trans and gender diverse children and adolescents* released by the Royal Children's Hospital in Melbourne (Telfer et al., 2017). In addition, guidelines and resources have been developed for specific healthcare professionals. For example, there are multiple guidelines and resources for psychologists and counsellors (e.g. American Psychological Association, 2015; Association for Lesbian, Gay, Bisexual, and Transgender Issues in Counseling, 2009; Australian Psychological Society, 2016), and a free module specifically developed for primary healthcare providers, including GPs (McNair, no date). Nonetheless, there is a pressing need for evidence-based practice guidelines for trans affirming care for young people. The present article makes an initial contribution to identifying what does and does not constitute such care.

Limitations

While this article contributes new knowledge relating to experiences of healthcare professionals amongst transgender young people and their parents, some limitations need to be acknowledged. This article draws on a pilot study with 10 parent/child dyads from two Australian states. In addition, the young people and their parents participated in dyad interviews and had attended gender clinics which suggests relatively high levels of family support. Finally, interviewing young people and their parent(s) together has possible limitations for what participants were willing to share in the interviews. However, this approach enabled young people and their parent(s) to build on each other's responses and provided support for participating.

Conclusion

In conclusion, we note that while the findings reported in this article highlight potential limitations to trans affirming care in Australia at present, there were also many examples of positive experiences. Young people appreciated the opportunity to be seen, heard, and affirmed. Participants especially valued healthcare professionals who went out of their way to provide affirming care. In regard to parents in particular, many participants appreciated opportunities to talk through their concerns, and believed that knowledgeable and affirming healthcare professionals were well placed to address such concerns. Even in cases where professionals were less knowledgeable than might be ideal, the opportunity to 'learn alongside one another' was valued by parents. These findings suggest that while there is still some way to go in terms of the provision of trans affirming care for transgender young people and their parents in Australia, there are many examples that suggest that such care provision is indeed possible. Recognising and transforming the conditions which reproduce cisgenderism in healthcare systems is essential for supporting this work.

Acknowledgements

The authors would like to thank the Canadian research team who developed the original project. They also thank the participants for sharing their experiences and views.

Disclosure statement

No potential conflict of interest was reported by the authors.

Funding

This study was funded by a Flinders University College of Education, Psychology and Social Work research grant. The second author was supported by an Australian Research Council Future Fellowship, FT130100087.

ORCID

Clare Bartholomaeus http://orcid.org/0000-0001-9843-8390
Damien W. Riggs http://orcid.org/0000-0003-0961-9099
Annie Pullen Sansfaçon http://orcid.org/0000-0003-2286-8997

References

American Psychological Association. (2015). *Guidelines for psychological practice with transgender and gender nonconforming people.*

Ansara, Y. G., & Hegarty, P. (2013). Misgendering in English language contexts: Applying non-cisgenderist methods to feminist research. *International Journal of Multiple Research Approaches, 7* (2), 160–177. doi:10.5172/mra.2013.7.2.160

Association for Lesbian, Gay, Bisexual, and Transgender Issues in Counseling. (2009). *Competencies for counseling with transgender clients.* Alexandria, VA: ALGBTIC.

Australian Psychological Society. (2016). *Information sheet: Australian Psychological Society recommends mental health practices that affirm transgender people's experiences.* Melbourne: Australian Psychological Society.

Bartholomaeus, C., & Riggs, D. W. (2020). Transgender and non-binary Australians' experiences with healthcare professionals in relation to fertility preservation. *Culture, Health & Sexuality, 22* (2), 129–145. doi:10.1080/13691058.2019.1580388

Blakey, A. G., & Treharne, G. J. (2019). Overcoming barriers to transgender healthcare education in Aotearoa New Zealand. *New Zealand Journal of Educational Studies, 54*(2), 357–366. doi:10.1007/s40841-019-00143-2

Braun, V., & Clarke, V. (2006). Using thematic analysis in psychology. *Qualitative Research in Psychology, 3*(2), 77–101. doi:10.1191/1478088706qp063oa

Carlile, A. (2020). The experiences of transgender and non-binary children and young people and their parents in healthcare settings in England, UK: Interviews with members of a family support group. *International Journal of Transgender Health, 21*(1), 16–32.

Chang, S. C., Singh, A. A., & dickey, l. m. (2018). *A clinician's guide to gender-affirming care: Working with transgender and gender nonconforming clients*. Oakland, CA: New Harbinger Publications.

Chen, D., Hidalgo, M. A., Leibowitz, S., Leininger, J., Simons, L., Finlayson, C., & Garofalo, R. (2016). Multidisciplinary care for gender-diverse youth: A narrative review and unique model of gender-affirming care. *Transgender Health, 1*(1), 117–123. doi:10.1089/trgh.2016.0009

Clark, B. A., Veale, J. F., Greyson, D., & Saewyc, E. (2018). Primary care access and foregone care: A survey of transgender adolescents and young adults. *Family Practice, 35*(3), 302–306. doi:10.1093/fampra/cmx112

Corliss, H. L., Belzer, M., Forbes, C., & Wilson, E. C. (2007). An evaluation of service utilization among male to female transgender youth: Qualitative study of a clinic-based sample. *Journal of LGBT Health Research, 3*(2), 49–61. doi:10.1300/J463v03n02_06

Eisenberg, M. E., McMorris, B. J., Rider, G. N., Gower, A. L., & Coleman, E. (2020). "It's kind of hard to go to the doctor's office if you're hated there." A call for gender-affirming care from transgender and gender diverse adolescents in the United States. *Health and Social Care in the Community, 28*(3), 1082–1089. doi:10.1111/hsc.12941

Goldenberg, T., Jadwin-Cakmak, L., Popoff, E., Reisner, S. L., Campbell, B. A., & Harper, G. W. (2019). Stigma, gender affirmation, and primary healthcare use among black transgender youth. *Journal of Adolescent Health, 65*(4), 483–490. doi:10.1016/j.jadohealth.2019.04.029

Gridley, S. J., Crouch, J. M., Evans, Y., Eng, W., Antoon, E., Lyapustina, M., … Breland, D. J. (2016). Youth and caregiver perspectives on barriers to gender-affirming health care for transgender youth. *Journal of Adolescent Health, 59*(3), 254–261. doi:10.1016/j.jadohealth.2016.03.017

Guss, C. E., Woolverton, G. A., Borus, J., Austin, S. B., Reisner, S. L., & Katz-Wise, S. L. (2019). Transgender adolescents' experiences in primary care: A qualitative study. *Journal of Adolescent Health, 65*(3), 344–349. doi:10.1016/j.jadohealth.2019.03.009

Heard, J., Morris, A., Kirouac, N., Ducharme, J., Trepel, S., & Wicklow, B. (2018). Gender dysphoria assessment and action for youth: Review of health care services and experiences of trans youth in Manitoba. *Paediatrics & Child Health, 23*(3), 179–184. doi:10.1093/pch/pxx156

Inwards-Breland, D. J., DiVall, S., Salehi, P., Crouch, J. M., Negaard, M., Lu, A., & Ahrens, K. R. (2019). Youth and parent experiences in a multidisciplinary gender clinic. *Transgender Health, 4*(1), 100–106. doi:10.1089/trgh.2018.0046

Kaltiala, R., Bergman, H., Carmichael, P., de Graaf, N. M., Rischel, K. E., Frisén, L., & Waehre, A. (2020). Time trends in referrals to child and adolescent gender identity services: A study in four Nordic countries and in the UK. *Nordic Journal of Psychiatry, 74*(1), 40–44. doi:10.1080/08039488.2019.1667429

McNair, R. (no date). *Primary healthcare for trans, gender diverse, and non-binary people*. Module. https://aelp.smartsparrow.com/v/open/f3xc2ipc.

Medico, D., Pullen Sansfaçon, A., Zufferey, A., Galantino, G., Bosom, M., & Suerich-Gulick, F. (2020). Pathways to gender affirmation in trans youth: A qualitative and participative study with youth and their parents. *Clinical Child Psychology and Psychiatry, 25*(4), 1002–1014. doi:10.1177/1359104520938427

Oliphant, J., Veale, J., Macdonald, J., Carroll, R., Johnson, R., Harte, M., … Bullock, J. (2018). *Guidelines for gender affirming healthcare for gender diverse and transgender children, young people and adults in Aotearoa, New Zealand*. Hamilton: Transgender Health Research Lab, University of Waikato.

Pullen Sansfaçon, A., Medico, D., Suerich-Gulick, F., & Temple Newhook, J. (2020). "I knew that I wasn't cis, I knew that, but I didn't know exactly": Gender identity development, expression and affirmation in youth who access gender affirming medical care. *International Journal of Transgender Health, 21*(3), 307–320. doi:10.1080/26895269.2020.1756551

Pullen Sansfaçon, A., Temple-Newhook, J., Suerich-Gulick, F., Feder, S., Lawson, M. L., Ducharme, J., & on behalf of the Stories of Gender-Affirming Care Team. (2019). The experiences of gender diverse and trans children and youth considering and initiating medical interventions in Canadian gender-affirming speciality clinics. *International Journal of Transgenderism, 20*(4), 371–387. doi:10.1080/15532739.2019.1652129

Riggs, D. W., Bartholomaeus, C., & Pullen Sansfaçon, A. (2020). 'If they didn't support me, I most likely wouldn't be here': Transgender young people and their parents negotiating medical treatment in Australia. *International Journal of Transgender Health, 21*(1), 3–15. doi:10.1080/15532739.2019.1692751

Riggs, D. W., Coleman, K., & Due, C. (2014). Healthcare experiences of gender diverse Australians: A mixed-methods, self-report survey. *BMC Public Health, 14*, 230–235. doi:10.1186/1471-2458-14-230

shuster, s. m. (2016). Uncertain expertise and the limitations of clinical guidelines in transgender healthcare. *Journal of Health and Social Behavior, 57*(3), 319–332. doi:10.1177/0022146516660343

Strauss, P., Cook, A., Winter, S., Watson, V., Wright Toussaint, D., & Lin, A. (2017). *Trans pathways: The mental health experiences and care pathways of trans young people.* Perth: Telethon Kids Institute.

Telfer, M., Tollit, M., & Feldman, D. (2015). Transformation of health-care and legal systems for the transgender population: The need for change in Australia. *Journal of Paediatrics and Child Health, 51*(11), 1051–1053. doi:10.1111/jpc.12994

Telfer, M., Tollit, M., Pace, C., & Pang, K. (2017). *Australian standards of care and treatment guidelines: For trans and gender diverse children and adolescents.* Melbourne: The Royal Children's Hospital.

Temple Newhook, J., Benson, K., Bridger, T., Crowther, C., & Sinnott, R. (2018). The TransKidsNL study: Healthcare and support needs of transgender children, youth, and families on the island of Newfoundland. *Canadian Journal of Community Mental Health, 37*(2), 13–28. doi:10.7870/cjcmh-2018-009

Tollit, M. A., Feldman, D., McKie, G., & Telfer, M. M. (2019). Patient and parent experiences of care at a pediatric gender service. *Transgender Health, 3*(1), 251–256. doi:10.1089/trgh.2018.0016

World Professional Association for Transgender Health. (2011). *Standards of care for the health of transsexual, transgender, and gender nonconforming people, 7th version.*

Not your unicorn: trans dating app users' negotiations of personal safety and sexual health

Kath Albury, Christopher Dietzel, Tinonee Pym, Son Vivienne and Teddy Cook

ABSTRACT

This article reflects on 14 Australian trans dating app users' accounts of feeling safer (and less safe) when using apps, as well as their experiences of sexual healthcare. We explore both app use and healthcare in the context of the interdisciplinary field of 'digital intimacies', considering the ways that digital technologies and cultures of technological use both shape and are shaped by broader professional and cultural norms relating to sexuality and gender. Drawing on Preciado's [(2013). *Testo junkie: Sex, drugs and biopolitics in the pharmacopornographic era*. The Feminist Press] framework of 'pharmacopornographisation', the analysis aims to contextualise participants' experiences of being 'seen' and 'known' by health professionals and other app users. Our findings indicate that both dating apps and sexual health services rely on reductive systems of sorting and categorisation that reinforce binary understandings of genders and sexualities in order to facilitate data management and information sharing practices. Yet these same sorting and filtering technologies can also help trans app users avoid harassment, form intimate connections and seek appropriate healthcare.

Since the mid 2000s, dating apps have become increasingly popular technologies for meeting and chatting to potential sexual and/or romantic partners. As Preciado (2013) has observed, the fields of sexual and reproductive medicine, sexology and pharmacology have developed alongside the proliferation of sexual technologies that primarily aim to enhance or promote sexual desire and pleasures. Drawing on Foucault's (1977, 1979) historical discussions of biopower, and de Lauretis' theorisation of 'technologies of gender' (1987), Preciado proposes a framework of 'pharmacopornographisation' as a means of understanding the ways that gender and sexuality become 'knowable' through a combination of embodied and technological practices. Preciado's account of the co-evolution of popular visual representations of sexuality and gender, and bio-medical and psychoanalytic understandings of 'normal' bodies, allow us to consider the ways that binary understandings of gender have been 'hard-wired' into both clinical settings and dating app technologies. This framework offers a useful lens for reflecting on trans people's experiences of both dating apps and sexual health services, particularly in relation to the tensions that arise in spaces where gender and sexuality are made 'visible' through practices such as sexual history-taking and diagnostic drop-down menus (in the space of healthcare), and through practices of self-disclosure on dating apps. In these spaces, sexuality and gender are classified and understood in ways that can simultaneously offer opportunities for care and intimacy, *and* restrict trans people's self-determination and safety.

This article is grounded in the emergent field of 'digital intimacies' (Burgess, Cassidy, Duguay, & Light, 2016; Dobson, Carah, & Robards, 2018); an interdisciplinary space that explores sexuality, gender and intimate relationships in the context of digital technologies (such as mobile phones) and digitally mediated settings (such as social media platforms and dating apps). While our discussion is necessarily limited in scale and scope, we deliberately seek to move beyond the risk-focused approach to app use that often characterises both popular conversations and public health communication (Albury, McCosker, Pym, & Byron, 2020). Instead, we explore both the opportunities and limitations that trans dating app users may encounter, asking 1) which aspects of app use contribute to users feeling safer, or less safe on apps; and 2) what would trans app users like health service providers to know about their experiences of sexual health care?

To this end, we reflect on qualitative workshops and interviews with 14 trans dating app users in New South Wales and Victoria (Australia). Our recruitment material invited 'trans, including gender diverse and non-binary, people' to share their experiences of app use. Where participants were cited directly, we have used their self-nominated gender description, and in other places we have used the term 'trans people' to describe our participants as an overall group. Trans people's qualitative accounts of dating app use – and experiences of sexual healthcare – are explored in the context of recent literature addressing the ways that digital media platform design, digital cultures of use, sexual health research and clinical practices may all impose limiting understandings of gender on their users. These experiences are not universally negative, however, with participants reporting multiple occasions where app design and infrastructures have facilitated safe and pleasurable connections with others. Drawing on participants' accounts of feeling safer (and less safe) when using apps – as well as their experiences of sexual healthcare – we consider the ways that normative assumptions around the 'knowability' of sexuality and gender impact trans people's experiences of both dating and healthcare, in order to suggest some strategies for health service providers seeking to better support them.

Background

Technologies of sex, sexuality and gender

Cultural theorist Paul Preciado links the twentieth century mainstreaming and popularisation of commercial and amateur pornography that made sex and gender 'visible' in new ways with the parallel mainstreaming and normalisation of pharmaceutical technologies that enhance or optimise users' appearance – and experience – in relation to both sexuality and gender. In his book *Testo Junkie* (2013), Preciado plots the progression of what Foucault has termed 'regimes of truth' in relation to sexuality and gender in the 19th and twentieth century. Drawing on de Lauretis' theorisations of cinema as a 'technology of gender' (1987), Preciado explores the relationship between the rise of new photographic and cinematic technologies, and the development of both bio-medical and psychoanalytic understandings of 'normal' gender and sexuality. While other scholars (such as Irvine, 1990) have explored the relationship between early psychoanalytic and sexological research and the emergence of photographic and cinematic pornography (and other forms of sex work); Preciado extends his discussion to consider the parallel development of bio-medical research into testosterone and estrogen, and the subsequent commercialisation of hormone therapies for both trans and cis people (2013, p. 388). He proposes the term 'pharmacopornographisation' as a means of theorising the complex 'network of power, knowledge and capital' (2013, p. 165) that is evident both within bio-medical assertions regarding the 'truth' of bodies and hormones; and within fetishised and/or commercialised representations of sexuality and gender in visual popular culture.

As he has more recently explained it, Preciado's framework of the pharmacopornographic extends Foucault's notions of biopower and biopolitics to incorporate recent technological developments of late-modernity, including the emergence of digital media technologies (Preciado, 2020). In this context, it is possible to understand a range of what Preciado terms the 'microprostheses and technologies of digital surveillance' – including Viagra, amyl nitrate, sex toys, lubricants, digital diagnostic platforms, social media platforms, self-help publications and tutorials, and photographic filtering software – through a 'pharmacopornographic' lens (Preciado, 2020). The conflation of 'pharma' and 'pornography' calls attention to the ways that both healthcare technologies and mediated representations of sexuality, gender and pleasure can be simultaneously understood as both commodities and expressions of care and intimacy.

While Preciado does not directly address dating app use, his accounts of the historical relationship between sexual and reproductive health research and clinical practice, and 'recreational' and/or eroticised practices of sexual representation, warn us against attempts to draw clear boundaries or hierarchies between 'medicalised' and 'sexualised' understandings of bodies, genders and sexualities. Further, just as researchers have drawn on popular and erotic texts to classify gender, the resulting biomedical 'technologies of gender' may also be translated into the design of social media platforms and apps. Clinical settings utilise technologies including medical intake forms and sexual history-taking protocols to sort and categorise clients according to expectations of 'risk' that are interwoven with historical expectations of gendered appearance and behaviour. Similarly, dating apps deploy technologies that invite users to categorise, filter and sort themselves – and others – in normatively gendered sexual and relational 'marketplaces'.

Trans people's experiences with dating apps

Like social media platforms, dating apps 'bake' gender into their design (Bivens & Haimson, 2016), in order to optimise their ability to aggregate, analyse (and market) user data (Albury et al., 2019; Szulc, 2019). Unsurprisingly, both dating apps and social media platforms have been subject to extensive critiques with respect to the ways that design features impose binary understandings of both gender and sexuality on their users, both via the drop-down menus and other interfaces used to build user profiles, and the facial and voice recognition systems used for security and identity-verification purposes (Ahmed, 2018; Ferris & Duguay, 2020; Scheuerman, Branham, & Hamidi, 2018, 2019).

Trans people's experiences of dating app use has been addressed within the fields of human–computer interaction, media and communications, gender studies and cultural studies. Significantly, this burgeoning field consistently reveals both positive and negative aspects of platform affordances and in-person experiences for trans users. These tensions and ambivalence are important when considering how health providers might speak to trans people about their sexual experiences, without assumptions or judgement. For example, Scheuerman et al. (2018) found that managing safety was a concern among all of their trans participants and that many had experienced technology-facilitated harm. Trans dating app users have reported being viewed as sexual objects (Lloyd & Finn, 2017) and being fetishised by others online in unwelcome ways (Platt & Bolland, 2017). Research has shown that trans people engaged in online dating have experienced high rates of violence and abuse, including physical violence, psychological violence, and sexual coercion, as well as technology-facilitated violence, such as receiving unwanted sexual images (Dank, Lachman, Zweig, & Yahner, 2014). Some may also experience additional violence because of their intersecting identities (Crenshaw, 1989) – that is, trans dating app users may feel less safe because of racism, ableism, ageism, and other discriminatory behaviour. Trans people also report that online spaces can offer them safe and comfortable ways to interact (Fox & Ralston, 2016) and can support trans users to explore 'identity work' and 'world-making' with peers (Schudson & Anders, 2019). Dating apps can be experienced as spaces for connecting with trans community, and identifying cis users who are respectful and informed about trans identities (Pym, Byron, & Albury, 2020).

A number of recent studies have considered the way trans dating app users navigate self representation in their profiles and chat practices, while also guarding their safety. In research by Scheim and colleagues (2019), gay, queer and bisexual trans men found that using apps and other platforms to meet cis men allowed them to 'bypass in-person disclosure' of their trans identity, and to pre-negotiate sexual activities and safer sex (2019, p. 578). However, 'balancing … potential pleasure against perceived risk' in relation to other app users' fetishistic, prescriptive or stigmatising attitudes commonly resulted in 'some degree of compromise or satisficing' (2019, pp. 579–582). Lloyd and Finn's (2017) research explores how trans women navigate transphobic, invalidating and fetishising interactions on Grindr (2017, pp. 162–4). While some of their interviewees distanced themselves from 'sexualised' self presentation to avoid being fetishised (2017, p. 163), others resisted the norms of cis femininity by deploying 'ambiguous authenticities' (2017, p. 165). For example, one participant acknowledged the 'validation' she received on apps and refused the regulatory force of aligning trans 'authenticity' with muted sexuality (2017, p. 165). The authors suggest that trans women's accounts demonstrate the limits of 'sexualisation' discourse, arguing that dating apps can offer users 'productive avenues for (re)working affirmative trans selfhoods and sexualities' (2017, p. 166).

Fernandez and Birnholtz (2019, p. 2) found that their interviewees preferred 'direct, proactive' disclosure of their trans identity on dating apps, as it felt safer to disclose with the physical distance of an app. Stating one's trans identity on a profile was considered to be 'less harmful' than more indirect forms of disclosure, insofar as it offered opportunities to filter out harassers, transphobes and unwelcome fetishists and to 'guard their time and emotional energy' (Fernandez & Birnholtz, 2019, pp. 10–12). Many sought 'a high level of certainty' that they were interacting with the right people, choosing to disclose in more than one part of their profile and in messaging (2019, p. 15). However, the cumulative experience of harassment following proactive disclosure led some participants to delete or avoid particular apps (2019, p. 14). Some interviewees preferred to post multiple photos that showed a range of aspects of their appearance and gender expression, or to emphasise their 'trans-ness' (2019, p. 12), while another preferred to disclose in chat, saying that disclosing on their profile put 'arbitrary' emphasis on their trans identity (2019, p. 13). In these examples, the authors highlight a 'tension between [participants'] desire for safety and a desire for authentic self-presentation.' (2019, p. 14).

Sexual health and dating apps

Research literature on dating apps in the field of sexual health spans the past decade, beginning with Grindr's release in 2009, followed by Tinder in 2012. A review of articles on sexual health and dating apps published between 2015 and 2018 ($n = 99$) found that the majority of this research focuses on STI/HIV prevention, mostly in regard to cis men who have sex with cis men (Albury et al., 2019). Although this review found an ongoing theme of 'sexual risk behaviours', there was little support for a connection of app use to sexual risk taking or STI/HIV transmissions. Trans people's sexual health in relation to dating apps and social media use has been addressed in a limited fashion, predominantly in studies focused on cis men who have sex with men (MSM) or LGBQ populations more broadly (Sun, Sutfin, Bachmann, Stowers, & Rhodes, 2018). This tendency is also reflected in more recent research, such as Macapagal et al.'s (2019) study of dating app use among 'sexual and gender minority adolescents assigned male at birth' with 6% of their participants 'gender nonconforming' and 'genderqueer' (and the remainder cis men), and Kesten et al.'s (2019) research on the 'acceptability and potential impact' of sexual health information delivered via dating apps for MSM, in which 2 out of 25 interviewees were trans.

Lesbian and queer women (cis and trans) do not appear at all in the 2015–2018 review sample (Albury et al., 2019). This is not limited to research on dating apps, but rather reveals a broader issue in health scholarship: as noted by Stardust, Cook, Hopkins, Gray, and Olsen (2017, p. 6), data collection in HIV research has consistently overlooked the many trans women who are lesbian or have sex with heterosexual men. HIV risk for trans men and non-binary people has also historically been inaccurately measured in HIV research due to 'inadequate gender-related questions in HIV diagnosis and notification process' (Stardust et al., 2017, p. 4). Further, public health and other disciplines have framed sexual health research around differences in sexuality rather than distinguishing between trans and cis people, or among gender diverse populations. Identity descriptions have not always encouraged or permitted trans people to identify themselves and, in some cases, confused gender with sexuality (e.g. Langenderfer-Magruder, Walls, Whitfield, Brown, & Barrett, 2016). Therefore, trans people may be included in 'MSM' literature, even if they are not identified.

In their survey of trans Australians, Callander et al. (2019, p. 9) found that 75.3% of respondents had used online services to seek sex and dating, and 'most felt that their gender was not respected by sex and dating web services or the people who use them.' Non-binary app users were the most common group to report feeling that dating apps and websites 'did not provide sufficient options to describe their genders' (Callander et al., 2019, p. 9). Callander et al.'s (2019, p. 13) report also found that 'failing to respect a patient's gender can discourage them from accessing important STI and HIV prevention and management strategies' – highlighting the impact that health practitioners can have on trans people's sexual health.

Methods

Our research findings are drawn from a larger project that aimed to promote dialogue between 18–35-year-old dating app users and sexual health organisations. To this end, we consulted with four project reference groups, including two app user groups, one mixed group of sexual health promotion professionals, sexuality educators and youth support workers, and one group of trans and gender-diverse health support workers. The project, an Australian Research Council partnership with two sexual health organisations, was approved by the Swinburne Human Research Ethics committee (SUHREC 2018/159), ACON's Research Ethics Review Committee (RERC 2018/12), and the Family Planning NSW Project Ethical Review Team (PERT 24). Our research differed from the public health studies outlined above in that it was primarily qualitative, and invited participants to define both 'sexual health' and 'safety' in their own terms. The analytical focus of this paper is trans app users' accounts of app use and sexual healthcare.

Participants were recruited via partner organisation mailing lists and social media accounts. Fourteen trans users of dating apps (median age 23.5) participated in interviews and workshops conducted from 2018–2020. Participants used different terms to describe their gender, including male, trans-male, non-binary, female, trans woman, genderqueer, non-binary transmasculine, agender and 'not that'. Sexual identities included gay, lesbian, straight, queer, bisexual, and pansexual. Cultural identities were self-described as Aboriginal/European, Anglo-Australian, Caucasian/Scottish, Caucasian, White/Pākeha, Australian, Maori/Australian, Aboriginal, and 'Mixed as.' We use self-nominated descriptors of sexuality and gender identities throughout this paper. All names are pseudonyms. Tinder was the dating app most used by participants, followed by Grindr. Other apps mentioned included HER, OKCupid, Bumble, and Scruff. Participants also reported using other social media and chat platforms for dating or hooking up, including Instagram, Tumblr, Reddit, Craigslist, Fetlife and Discord.

As Barker and colleagues (2012) observe, creative research methods (particularly visual methods) can offer opportunities for participants to express aspects of their lived experiences of sexuality and gender that may not emerge in more 'traditional' research settings. For this reason, we incorporated elements of creative and visual research methodologies into both research workshops and one-to-one interviews. Interviews were conducted via a modified 'media go-along" (Jørgensen, 2016), in which participants were invited to share their personal history of app use, and experiences of negotiating personal safety and sexual health on apps. Interviewees were invited to open any dating apps currently on their phones (without sharing their screens with the interviewer), and reflect on past interactions with other users, using their own app history as a visual prompt.

Workshop activities included drawing (and discussing) maps or timelines depicting all the apps and platforms participants had ever used for dating and hooking up, with attention to any interruptions or shifts in app use over time. Participants were also invited to share their 'top tips' for app use (in the style of an online dating advice article); and to design two alternative profiles for a hypothetical friend who had not previously used apps. The first profile contained elements that might signal a 'dateable/trustworthy' app-user, while the second profile was full of 'red flags', or signs the app user might be unsafe or untrustworthy. This design activity prompted extended discussions of the ways participants crafted their own profiles to promote safe, pleasurable encounters, and the ways they interpret others' profiles as more or less safe. At the close of the workshop, participants were invited to tell us what they wanted sexual health services to know about their experiences.

Interviews and workshops were facilitated by both trans and cis members of the research team. They were audio-recorded, transcribed and coded using Nvivo software by two cis researchers via a process of abductive analysis (Tavory & Timmermans, 2014), which combines inductive and deductive approaches. Prominent sub-themes identified included: developing confidence and establishing boundaries; filtering out deceptive users; experiences of harassment and abuse; navigating app infrastructures (regarding binary gender and sexuality categories); disclosure of trans status and educating cis users; and sexual health discussions both on apps and with health professionals. Following preliminary analyses, this article was co-authored by a team of trans and cis researchers, including two members of the trans project advisory group.

Trans people's experiences of dating apps

Feeling safer on dating apps

Eight participants discussed having felt unsafe or vulnerable to violence or harassment on apps or in meetups, with two commenting that this was under-acknowledged by cis friends. Nine participants described encountering app profiles or experiencing chats that were transphobic, biphobic, racist or discriminatory towards sex workers, and Stephen (27, bisexual, trans male) felt app developers should take a stronger stance in counteracting discriminatory attitudes on their platforms. Participants had a range of strategies for interpreting other users' profile information in order to screen out stigmatising, fetishising or discriminatory users.

Deceptive users and fake profiles were a concern for the majority of our participants, who discussed strategies for filtering these out by interpreting profile information and photos as well as navigating the chat/messaging process. For Blair (23, lesbian, female), this meant taking time to check whether a user's 'story' was consistent, and meeting only after a week or two of chat. Social media platforms – such as Instagram or Facebook – were an important avenue for establishing trust while dating, although participants used these in different ways.

Some felt more secure when they could access their match's social media accounts – for three of our participants, failure to move app-based chats to other social platforms was considered a 'red flag', or sign that the other user had malicious intent. This aligns with findings from other studies of contemporary digital intimacies which identify what Madianou and Miller (2013) have termed 'polymedia practices', in which app users connect across a range of social media platforms – including chat and picture-sharing platforms – to establish trust and negotiate safety within intimate relationships (Albury et al., 2019; Cassidy, 2018; Venema & Lobinger, 2017). However, some were wary about requests to move a conversation to social media too quickly (or at all), expressing privacy concerns.

Three participants felt that app platforms offering formal identity verification (such as Bumble's blue check mark, which indicates the profile has been verified by a staff member) would help them to feel safer, but recognised the limitations for trans app users whose appearance may not match the app developer's understandings of 'appropriate' gendered presentation. Blair suggested it was a problem for trans users when app platforms instituted official identity verification, as they may not be out, and/or their appearance may alter as they affirm their gender. She initially used exclusively text-based platforms to avoid the issue of profile photos: 'I didn't want people to associate – because I wasn't out back then, if they saw me on a dating app – to realise that I was presenting as female and that I was trans.'

Two participants were also on the alert for 'chasers' – that is, app users (usually cis men) with a highly sexualised and fetishistic attraction to trans people. Avery (24, queer, 'not that') said, 'Anyone who approaches me for being gender non-conforming in any fucking way are usually fetishising that, and straight up that's a fuck no … keep chasers chasing.' Parker (22, straight, trans-male) noted that although some users attempt to deter 'chasers' in their profile text (i.e. 'not your unicorn'), they felt this strategy had limited efficacy. Experiences with cis men on apps were viewed as unsafe in a range of contexts. Three participants reported frequently encountering fake profiles (where photos or in-app chat signalled 'catfishing') on queer women's apps, or seeing cis men's profiles on mixed-gender apps when the user had elected not to be matched with men at all. Others had encounters with cis men on queer men's apps that they experienced as pushy, prescriptive, or aggressive.

Disclosing trans identity on apps

Participants discussed the challenges of disclosing trans and non-binary identities on apps, acknowledging that while placing the information upfront in a profile could filter out the wrong users, it could also render them vulnerable to intrusive questions and fetishisation. Experiences of disclosure varied widely, with some participants suggesting that the design of specific apps (and collective cultures of use) had a significant impact in this respect:

> My gender's more accessible because I've ticked the trans box on Grindr, but for Tinder that didn't come around for a very long time and with Tinder … most of them are generally cis-gender straight women and they're not really down for meeting a trans person. So I find that Grindr, people are more accepting of hooking up with a trans person. Yeah, because this app has always had the system there to identify as trans. (Quinn, 24, bisexual, male)

Alex (26, lesbian, non-binary) felt that identifying as 'non-binary' in their Pink Cupid profile was rejected by some lesbian cis women as 'high-maintenance' because it required dates to 'remember your pronouns'. Sam (23, pansexual, non-binary) had rarely had problems disclosing non-binary identity on HER, but cautioned that this was not necessarily evidence that trans people were welcome on the app: 'maybe people are less shook by a non-binary person than like a binary trans person' on that platform.

Participants also reported encountering transphobia in user profiles (e.g. 'cis4cis') as well as in chats. Max (23, queer, non-binary transmasculine) had encountered transphobic reactions from cis straight app users, and described switching between gender and sexuality categories regularly on Tinder to avoid them: 'if I'm showing myself as a man I'll only look at the [queer] men, and if I'm showing myself as a woman, I'll only look at the queer women.' A range of approaches were reported in terms of responding to cis app users asking intrusive questions about bodies and identities (both on apps and after meeting for dates in person). Four participants were strongly opposed to answering cis users' questions, feeling they should self-educate. However, Blair was happy to do this as she compared it to her own curiosity about other trans people's experiences. There was no consensus among participants regarding how to respond to trans app users' questions. Jesse (34, gay, male) specifically avoided in-app chats with other trans users who they felt were seeking information or social support. In contrast, Avery said they had directed a trans app user to trans-inclusive spaces and resources.

Despite the challenges outlined here, the majority of participants found their overall experiences with apps to be positive. For example, Quinn experienced Grindr as a space where they felt affirmed in their body and identity: 'There's always been a space for me on Grindr ... the acceptance of me is their attraction to men and I'm part of that.' The range in participants' experiences suggests that dating apps are spaces that hold potential for trans dating app users to feel more and/or less safe depending both on the app's technical infrastructure and the attitudes of fellow app-users.

Apps and sexual health

A number of participants said they wanted to receive information about sexual health and sexual health resources through apps. Since some apps already provide reminders about getting tested for STIs and HIV, participants felt it would be valuable for apps to be active in sexual health promotion more generally. Notably, they suggested incorporating pop-up notifications and links to community organisations, resources and information. Avery emphasised the importance of 'having a plan' in relation to sexual health on apps, and this included knowing in advance how to respond to slut-shaming or the use of stigmatising language around sexual health (e.g. 'clean') in app-based chats.

> 'Safe sex' was understood by participants to mean different things depending on context. For example, Tristan (32, bi, male) said that although he personally associated sexual health with regular HIV/STI testing, knowing his status, and using contraception, his own check-in app conversations prior to meeting up were limited to confirming a preference for condom use.

A number of participants observed that sexual health is discussed less frequently within the lesbian community than among gay men – and this was reflected in their experiences of using apps. Blair said that women might check in about STI status after getting to know one another better (she herself usually asked), but also thought that sexual health was viewed as less relevant for lesbians. Alex was frustrated that lesbians 'don't disclose things', however they felt that apps incorporating STI testing into profile fields would feel 'invasive' to app users:

> I find the lesbian community don't really open up about sexual health a lot. Within the apps it's not talked about. I'm quite an open person so I usually do ask these things and people sometimes will be like, 'Oh, this is a bit invasive' and I'm just like, 'Well, no not really it's just your sexual health. It's me caring about myself and caring about you.'

Sam noted that although the app HER had a community forum which sometimes hosts discussions about sexual health, they felt that few users engaged with these discussions. Quinn said they list 'negative' on their profile and are on PrEP and have regular tests. However, as they did not use condoms and have experienced repeated problems with the supply of their preferred hormones, they sometimes worry about pregnancy when having sex with cis men.

Tristan was new to dating cis men and felt ill-informed about sexual health in this context, and he was concerned that raising the topic on apps would compound his concerns about rejection:

> I worry about it in terms of just being trans. Just from the aspect of being rejected as well. Yeah, I worry about sexual health on Grindr because I don't really know much about the gay community in terms of guys because I used to only be interested in women before.

While Tristan sought more sexual health advice on apps (in the form of 'top tips'), others felt that apps like Grindr shared too much of this kind of content.

What do app users want health professionals to know?

Participants had mixed experiences of discussing sexual health with general practitioners (GPs) and other health professionals. Many were open to being asked about their sexual history, provided that the information was necessary in context and assumptions were not made about them. Tristan believed it was important for GPs to ask questions about partners and sexual practices, but it could be 'invasive' and 'creepy' if the questions did not seem relevant to the consultation. Trust in a doctor was important in feeling that questions were asked in good faith, and trans-friendly clinics were an important aspect of this.

A trans-affirming GP was also thought to be more likely to offer useful prompts for questions patients might not think to disclose themselves, but which were relevant to further health advice. For example, Tristan mentioned his doctor asking if he had developed a sexual interest in men, which he found helpful 'because people don't always disclose stuff … and it's easier when they're asked directly.' Blair felt that she lacked knowledge about women's sexual health, and suggested health professionals could check in to make sure trans patients and their sexual partners were aware of what their concerns should be. However, three participants reported feeling judged or 'put in a box' by health professionals' assumptions about their gender, sexual identity and practices. Parker said:

> I walk in and you've already made up your mind about what I need … don't question my sexuality. I had a doctor do that to me … he was like, 'So what made you think you liked women?' I was like, what the fuck?

Avery suggested that health professionals could offer trans patients more agency by asking them for their safe sex plan at the outset, and then filling in the gaps by asking additional questions if needed. They added that professionals should avoid expecting trans patients to explain sexual practices that the practitioner may be unfamiliar with, and should take more initiative in self-educating about the associated risks of a range of practices.

Within our broader study, app users of diverse sexualities and genders suggested that sexual healthcare professionals were often not well-informed of the 'ordinary' role that dating and hook-up apps play in contemporary cultures of sexuality and friendship. This suggestion was confirmed by participants in our professional reference groups, who agreed that while staff in LGBTQ+ community health services were often familiar with the everyday aspects of app use, this was not universally the case in more generalist settings. This suggests that trans app users attending general practices are more likely to encounter service providers who are less aware of the ways sexual health negotiations could be both facilitated and discouraged by the specific cultures of use and technical infrastructures on diverse apps.

Discussion and conclusions

As noted by Callander et al. (2019), dating app design, sexual health surveillance and reporting practices can all serve as 'technologies of gender', imposing binary gender categories on trans people. Within dating app cultures, users are often assumed to be cis by default. Further, while popular apps such as Tinder or Grindr allow users to choose non-binary options for themselves (while constructing their profile), searching and matching are limited to 'men', 'women', or 'both'. This places an obligation on trans app users to make a difficult choice: Do they disclose their 'difference' in their public profiles (and risk unwanted approaches and/or intrusive questioning by transphobic, predatory, fetishising or 'curious' individuals)? Or do they withhold information, and risk being accused of 'deception' by transphobic or trans-exclusionary cis users who assumed they were matched with another cis person?

We note that our study focused primarily on trans people's in-app experiences and did not examine the broader sexual health issues they might confront when dating. Further, our relatively small sample size could be improved upon in order to capture a wider range of trans app users' experiences. Our findings further suggest there may be significantly different approaches and concerns with regard to both personal safety and sexual health expressed by trans users of apps focused on 'men seeking men' or 'women seeking women', as opposed to 'straight' apps.

As noted above, app-users who identify as non-binary, agender, genderqueer or gender-fluid may also experience specific safety concerns in relation to the binary nature of dating apps' (and social media platforms') interfaces and sorting/filtering mechanisms. As Bivens' (2015) analysis of back-end coding of gender on Facebook revealed:

> deep in the database, users who select custom gender options are re-coded—without their knowledge—back into a binary/other classification system . . . . [Facebook's] custom gender project offers the illusion of inclusion since surface changes to profile pages mask the binary regulation that continues underneath, at a deeper level of the software. (Bivens, 2015, p. 885)

Further, for some of our participants, their experiences of using apps and attending to their healthcare needs converged in ways that could easily be interpreted via Preciado's lens of the 'pharmacopornographic'. For example, Quinn's experiences of both sexual health and app use were influenced by their use of 'MSM' dating apps in which it was easy for them to negotiate the kinds of sex they desired by openly disclosing their use of PrEP, but more difficult for them to ask questions about sexual health more generally, or discuss their concerns regarding contraception. Other participants reported similar frustrations in sexual health settings, where health professionals mis-gendered them, or conflated their gender expression or gender identity with their sexual identity or preferred sexual behaviours. In these cases, the burden falls on the trans person to either assume the responsibility of educating the health professional, or remain silent, and risk receiving inadequate or unsatisfactory levels of care or information.

In a 2020 reflection on the ways the contemporary entanglement of digital technologies, healthcare, gender and sexuality might be understood via a 'pharmacopornographic' lens, Preciado argued for a deeper consideration of the 'management and production of the body as well as … the political technologies that produce sexual subjectivity within this new configuration of power and knowledge' (np). Within our study, we see pharmacopornographisation playing out in a number of ways. Both dating apps and health services rely on reductive systems of sorting and categorisation that reinforce binary understandings of genders and sexualities in order to facilitate data management and information sharing practices. Yet these same sorting and filtering technologies can also help trans app users avoid harassment, form intimate connections and seek appropriate healthcare.

We note that there was little consensus among trans people in our study on the practices or platforms they experienced as positive or negative, with many people noting their own ambivalence or complicity and observing that some behaviours and/or platform infrastructures can have simultaneously positive and negative consequences. Participants reported similar ambivalence in regard to sexual healthcare settings, where their sexuality and gender were challenged or subjected to 'excessive' questioning. At the same time, practices of self-disclosure – both on dating apps and within medical settings – were seen as valuable, necessary and even desirable for some. This reflects the deliberate ambiguity evident within Preciado's theorisations of both sexual popular culture and the medicalisation of sexuality and gender, in which he emphasised the ways that even the most 'commodified' or 'objectifying' technologies of gender can be deployed strategically and productively by trans people.

As noted above, two participants explicitly said they needed more sexual health information, and wanted to access this both on apps and in healthcare settings. As with dating apps, participants were willing to enter into imperfect sexual healthcare cultures that might not fully 'see' or 'know' them, but they wanted to be recognised and affirmed in these spaces in ways that did not rely on normative assumptions, stigma or fetishisation.

Both dating apps and sexual health research have drawn on systems of gender classification that construct gendered subjects through a simultaneously technologised and fetishised 'pharmacopornographic' lens. Unsurprisingly, our participants reported experiences of sexual healthcare in which seemingly neutral practices (such as questions regarding sexual histories) placed trans people in the position of having to defend, justify or explain their sexualities and genders in ways that were experienced as similarly insensitive and intrusive. We do not conclude, however, that trans app users in our study do not want to discuss sexual health with medical practitioners; rather, they want to have these discussions in informed, trans-affirming contexts.

Disclosure statement

No potential conflict of interest was reported by the author(s).

Funding

This work was supported by Australian Research Council: [Grant Number LP160101687]; Mitacs.

ORCID

Kath Albury http://orcid.org/0000-0001-9043-8126
Tinonee Pym http://orcid.org/0000-0001-6731-4475

References

Ahmed, A. A. (2018). Trans competent interaction design: A qualitative study on voice, identity, and technology. *Interacting with Computers*, *30*(1), 53–71.

Albury, K., Byron, P., McCosker, A., Pym, T., Walshe, J., Race, K., … Dietzel, C. (2019). *Safety, risk and wellbeing on dating apps: Final report*. Swinburne University of Technology. doi:10.25916/5dd324c1b33bb.

Albury, K., McCosker, A., Pym, T., & Byron, P. (2020). Dating apps as public health 'problems': Cautionary tales and vernacular pedagogies in news media. *Health Sociology Review*, *29*(3), 232–248. doi:10.1080/14461242.2020.1777885

Barker, M., Richards, C., & Bowes-Catton, H. (2012). Visualizing experience: Using creative research methods with members of sexual and gender communities. In C. N. Phellas (Ed.), *Researching non-heterosexual sexualities* (pp. 57–80). Farnham: Ashgate.

Bivens, R. (2015). The gender binary will not be deprogrammed: Ten years of coding gender on Facebook. *New Media & Society*, *19*(6), 880–898.

Bivens, R., & Haimson, O. L. (2016). Baking gender into social media design: How platforms shape categories for users and advertisers. *Social Media + Society*, *2*(4), 1–12.

Burgess, J., Cassidy, E., Duguay, S., & Light, B. (2016). Making digital cultures of gender and sexuality with social media. *Social Media + Society*, *2*(4), 1–4.

Callander, D., Wiggins, J., Rosenberg, S., Cornelisse, V. J., Duck-Chong, E., Holt, M., … Cook, T. (2019). *The 2018 Australian trans and gender diverse sexual health survey: Report of findings*. Sydney: The Kirby Institute, UNSW.

Cassidy, E. (2018). *Gay men, identity and social media: A culture of participatory reluctance*. New York: Routledge.

Crenshaw, K. (1989). Demarginalizing the intersection of race and sex: Black feminist critique of antidiscrimination doctrine, feminist theory and antiracist politics. *University of Chicago Legal Forum*, *1989*(1), 139–168.

Dank, M., Lachman, P., Zweig, J. M., & Yahner, J. (2014). Dating violence experiences of lesbian, gay, bisexual, and transgender youth. *Journal of Youth and Adolescence*, *43*, 846–857.

De Lauretis, T. (1987). *Technologies of gender*. Indiana University Press.

Dobson, A. S., Carah, N., & Robards, B. (2018). Digital intimate publics and social media: Towards theorising public lives on private platforms. In A. S. Dobson, N. Carah, & B. Robards (Eds.), *Digital intimate publics and social media* (pp. 3–27). Palgrave Macmillan.

Fernandez, J. R., & Birnholtz, J. (2019). 'I don't want them to not know': Investigating decisions to disclose transgender identity in dating platforms. *Proceedings of the ACM on Human-Computer Interaction, 3*, 1–21.

Ferris, L., & Duguay, S. (2020). Tinder's lesbian digital imaginary: Investigating (im)permeable boundaries of sexual identity on a popular dating app. *New Media & Society, 22*(3), 489–506.

Foucault, Michel. (1975). *Discipline and punish: The birth of the prison* (Alan Sheridan, Trans.; 1st ed.). (1977 first US ed)

Foucault, Michel. (1978). *The history of sexuality volume 1: An introduction* [trans. Robert Hurley] Pantheon (original French 1st ed. 1976)

Fox, J., & Ralston, R. (2016). Queer identity online: Informal learning and teaching experiences of LGBTQ individuals on social media. *Computers in Human Behavior, 65*, 635–642.

Irvine, J. (1990). *Disorders of desire: Sex and gender in modern American sexology*. Philadelphia: Temple University Press.

Jørgensen, K. M. (2016). The media go-along: Researching mobilities with media at hand. *MedieKultur: Journal of Media and Communication Research, 60*, 31–49.

Kesten, J. M., Dias, K., Burns, F., Crook, P., Howarth, A., Mercer, C. M., ... Weatherburn, P. (2019). Acceptability and potential impact of delivering sexual health promotion information through social media and dating apps to MSM in England: A qualitative study. *BMC Public Health, 19*(1236), 1–9.

Langenderfer-Magruder, L., Walls, N. E., Whitfield, D. L., Brown, S. M., & Barrett, C. M. (2016). Partner violence victimization among lesbian, gay, bisexual, transgender, and queer youth: Associations among risk factors. *Child and Adolescent Social Work Journal, 33*(1), 55–68.

Lloyd, C. E., & Finn, M. D. (2017). Authenticity, validation and sexualisation on Grindr: An analysis of trans women's accounts. *Psychology & Sexuality, 8*(1–2), 158–169.

Macapagal, K., Kraus, A., Moskowitz, D. A., & Birnholtz, J. (2019). Geosocial networking application use, characteristics of app-met sexual partners, and sexual behavior among sexual and gender minority adolescents assigned male at birth. *The Journal of Sex Research, 57*(8), 1078–1087.

Madianou, M., & Miller, D. (2013). Polymedia: Towards a new theory of digital media in interpersonal communication. *International Journal of Cultural Studies, 16*(2), 169–187.

Platt, L. F., & Bolland, K. S. (2017). Trans* partner relationships: A qualitative exploration. *Journal of GLBT Family Studies, 13*(2), 163–185.

Preciado, P. (2020). Learning from the virus. *ArtForum*. Retrieved from https://www.artforum.com/print/202005/paul-b-preciado-82823.

Preciado, P. B. (2013). *Testo junkie: Sex, drugs and biopolitics in the pharmacopornographic era*. New York: The Feminist Press.

Pym, T., Byron, P., & Albury, K. (2020). 'I still want to know they're not terrible people': Negotiating 'queer community' on dating apps. *International Journal of Cultural Studies*. doi:10.1177/1367877920959332

Scheim, A. I., Adam, B. D., & Marshall, Z. (2019). Gay, bisexual, and queer trans men navigating sexual fields. *Sexualities, 22*(4), 566–586.

Scheuerman, M. K., Branham, S. M., & Hamidi, F. (2018). Safe spaces and safe places: Unpacking technology-mediated experiences of safety and harm with transgender people. *Proceedings of the ACM on Human-Computer Interaction, 2*(CSCW), 1–27.

Scheuerman, M. K., Paul, J. M., & Brubaker, J. R. (2019). How computers see gender: An evaluation of gender classification in commercial facial analysis and image labeling services. *Proceedings of the ACM on Human-Computer Interaction, 3*, 1–33.

Schudson, Z., & Anders, S. (2019). 'You have to coin new things': Sexual and gender identity discourses in asexual, queer, and/or trans young people's networked counterpublics. *Psychology & Sexuality, 10*(4), 354–368.

Stardust, Z., Cook, T., Hopkins, L., Gray, J., & Olsen, K. (2017). *Effective and meaningful inclusion of trans and gender diverse people in HIV prevention*. Sydney: ACON and PASH.tm.

Sun, C. J., Sutfin, E., Bachmann, L. H., Stowers, J., & Rhodes, S. D. (2018). Comparing men who have sex with men and transgender women who use Grindr, other similar social and sexual networking apps, or no social and sexual networking apps: Implications for recruitment and health promotion. *Journal of AIDS & Clinical Research*, *9*(2), 757.

Szulc, L. (2019). Profiles, identities, data: Making abundant and anchored selves in a platform society. *Communication Theory*, *29*(3), 257–276.

Tavory, I., & Timmermans, S. (2014). *Abductive analysis: Theorizing qualitative research.* Chicago: University of Chicago Press.

Venema, R., & Lobinger, K. (2017). "And somehow it ends up on the Internet." agency, trust and risks in photo-sharing among friends and romantic partners. *First Monday*, *22*(7). Retrieved from https://firstmonday.org/ojs/index.php/fm/article/view/7860.

Transgender health: on a world scale

Raewyn Connell

ABSTRACT
Understanding transgender health on a world scale requires an adequate conceptualisation of gender as an embodied social structure, and an awareness of imbalances in the global economy of knowledge. Four major clusters of health issues are identified for trans groups in the majority, postcolonial world: staying alive in the face of violence and disease, keeping a trans life afloat in practice, facing pressures including rising populism, and making transitions work. Familiar models of professional health care are not adequate to these issues across much of the world; social action and organising are required.

Gender and knowledge about gender

To think clearly about health for transgender and gender diverse people, we need to pay attention to the realities of gender. When a framing concept is offered in the health literature about these groups, it is most often a simple idea of gender as a personal 'identity'. Trans identities are presumed to contrast with a dominant binary system of norms where identities must be either man or woman, girl or boy. Identities are recognisable as trans/gender-diverse if they (a) lack a conventional alignment with male or female bodies (i.e. are not cisgender), or (b) are fluid, ambivalent, undecidable, or opposed to the binary. In any of these cases, it is an individual identity that is at stake. On the basis of this conception, the literature builds notions of individual rights to expression of personal identity. Treatment practices are criticised for violation of these rights, and critiques of the dominance of binary gender discourse are built.

There is a paradox here. The 'personal identity' framework achieves the remarkable feat of *de-gendering* the language that is used to talk about people for whom gender is a matter of great importance. When the analysis is conducted through terms like 'trans individuals', 'non-normative identities', 'trans*', or 'cis people', it has effectively sidelined gender relations. Gender terms like 'patriarchy', 'rape culture', 'perinatal mortality rates', 'protest masculinity' or 'sister' seem to go missing. (They may appear later, however, in empirical details.)

I think it is important to bring gender solidly back into the picture. This does not mean asserting a 'binary'. As a matter of fact, gender structures have never been binary. They are *much* more complicated. There is a mass of social, ethnographic and psychological research documenting the multiple forms of masculinities, femininities and gender configurations that are neither, and – also important – the divisions and contradictions within them. Socially recognised gender divisions change with age, and vary between ethnic and religious groups, regions, industries and whole cultures. Kinship structures often involve very complex differentiations.

How do we know relations or practices are gender relations or practices? All of the patterns just mentioned have some connection with human biological reproduction. Our method of reproduction is sexual, combining genetic information from male and female bodies (until the geneticists take a few more scary steps!). The connection of a social relationship with reproduction may be close or remote, and it may be symbolic or mediated. But that connection is what defines *gender* relations as distinct from other patterns of social relationship such as class.

Gender is fundamentally a matter of social relationships, which are connected with (but *not* determined by) that reproductive arena. Gender relations and structures include, as well as discourse and identity, *economic relations* such as gender divisions of labour, *power relations* such as control of the means of violence, and *affective relationships* such as patterns of love and hatred (for this social framework see Connell, 2021). Through these dimensions we define aggregates of people that we name in gender terms (as boys, mothers, effeminate men, etc.), forming the familiar landscape of our gendered social life. Individual gender attribution concerns affiliation with such groups in relations of solidarity, recognition, exclusion and so forth. The process of claiming and enacting membership and affiliation appears constantly in the narratives of groups regarded as 'trans' – and for other groups too. As Simone de Beauvoir famously remarked, 'One is not born, but rather becomes, a woman'. She did not have trans women in mind at the time.

Finally, a crucial fact. The majority of people to whom a term like 'trans and gender diverse' might apply do not live in rich countries of the global North, nor rich settler-colonial countries like Australia. They live in central and south America, sub-Saharan Africa, Muslim-majority countries, south, south-east, and east Asia, and the Pacific: the majority world. However, the great bulk of the health-related research literature about trans and gender diverse people is conducted in the global North, and is about people in the global North. Or if it is done elsewhere, it uses concepts, methods and citations derived from the global North.

This imbalance is entirely familiar in health sciences. Indeed it is endemic in the modern global economy of knowledge (Collyer, Connell, Maia, & Morrell, 2019). Any field of the human sciences structured this way is liable to miss very important matters. I believe this has happened in the field of trans health. To correct it, we need to think about trans health on a world scale. To do that – as in any field of the human sciences (Connell, 2007; Reiter, 2018) we need to reverse the usual priorities, and give primary attention to experience and information from the global South.

Major health problems faced by 'trans and gender diverse' groups

The observations that follow are based on meetings with trans support groups in seven countries of the postcolonial world, rich and poor, and on a search for literature about the experience of transitions (of various kinds and degrees) in the majority world. I suggest there are four principal groups of health issues.

Staying alive

Some years ago I was talking with a trans support group at a coffee shack in Costa Rica, a small and beautiful country of central America. In the course of a long conversation we somehow got to the topic of how long we expected to live. Consensus in the local group was that trans women, including *travestis*, could expect about 32 years of life. But in a next-door country, where death squads were operating, they could expect less. I was suddenly conscious that I was the oldest present, by far.

Significant numbers of trans women work in the sex trade, and in this industry occupational health and safety take a distinctive form. Sex workers are vulnerable to violence from clients, neighbours, police, and industry bosses. Natatxa Carreras Sendra (2009) recorded, in a group of about 45 *vestidas* in street sex work in Puebla (Mexico), six deaths by murder and one probable murder within 15 years. A study of trans sex workers in northern Mexico reports a high level of police harassment and many arrests: 83% of *travesti* and transgender sex workers had been gaoled at some point, compared with 7% of sex workers who were not trans (Castillo, Gudelia, Gómez, & Rosas Solís, 2010). Prison is an exceptionally dangerous environment for any feminine trans group, with the risk of rape, bashings and suicide. We know that incarceration rates are appallingly high for Indigenous communities in settler-colonial contexts. In a widely known case in Australia a decade ago, an Indigenous trans woman, Veronnica Baxter, was arrested and held in a men's prison. Six days later she was found dead, apparently after making emergency calls from her cell that were either not answered or not recorded. The death was recorded as suicide.

In a number of regions there are threats from vigilantes, state-backed death squads, or armed para-statal groups. Trans groups are targeted along with homeless people, homosexual men and other marginalised groups. Violence of this kind is euphemised as 'social cleansing', *limpieza social*, in Central and South America, the regions where it is best documented (DFensor, 2012; Serrano-Amaya, 2018). It certainly occurs in other regions too. An international review of research (Kidd & Witten, 2007) found hate crimes against transgender groups to be a global phenomenon. It is often unclear whether violence occurred because of being trans, or being a woman, or being a sex worker, but whatever the reason, killings occur.

Violence has a broader health downstream: injuries, disability and stress. Poor housing and poor nutrition mean vulnerability to infectious diseases such as tuberculosis. In sex work, trans workers often have limited chances of negotiating safe sex: Carreras Sendra's study found that 16 of her group of *vestidas* died from AIDS. Occupational health and safety in such a context is not great.

Keeping afloat

Crowded housing, entry to sex work, and vulnerability to social cleansing are all linked to poverty. Poverty, in turn, is a likely consequence of being thrown out of home, driven out of school, or sacked from a job when transition becomes visible; these are commonplace items in trans women's stories. We know, from a massive body of research in public health – including the famous report of the Commission on Social Determinants of Health (WHO, 2008) – that class situation is correlated with many forms of illness and trauma. Further, poverty and wealth strongly affect access to health services. In the absence of a well-resourced public health system, if you do not have money you cannot get specialist treatment, sterile equipment or expensive materials. In many places there is a street trade in hormones. There are no quality controls in the street.

Losing one's income or family home means surviving in a housing crisis. The result may be living on the streets, living in very cheap apartments or short-term hotels. A constructive solution is to form a local network or communal housing, as one finds among *hijra* in India (Reddy, 2006) and in trans groups' squats in Brazil. Homelessness may also push towards migration. Migration from region to region or across international borders seems a very common experience for trans women, sometimes, as Amy Ritterbusch (2016) puts it, at gunpoint. Migration often provides no relief from insecurity, either economic or physical, especially when moving between different languages and legal regimes (Namaste, 2015).

These problems are reasonably common across the global South, and they point to requirements for effective support and organisation. An excellent example is provided by the *Centro de Atención Integral a la Diversidad Sexual y de Género* in Martires, an inner-city area in Colombia (Alcaldía Mayor de Bogotá, 2014). CAIDS was set up in 2014 in a dangerous neighbourhood that is a centre of the sex trade. Its director is a highly capable trans woman; its participants mostly work in the sex trade locally. The building has a restaurant; it provides a point of connection, a place where stories are exchanged, deaths are mourned, and new possibilities are seen. CAIDS provides meeting rooms, socio-legal counselling, an art room with video facilities, and certificate courses in dressmaking and hairdressing (jobs actually open to trans women) run by the city's technical education department. It thus offers multiple services meeting different needs to make trans lives viable.

Pressure

Poverty and displacement trigger a search for income, often in occupational niches. Theatre is a traditional context for *kathoey* lives in Thailand. Hairdressing and beauty parlours are relatively open in Colombia and in Brazil (Serrano-Amaya, 2018; de Souza & de Carrieri, 2015), and doubtless in other countries. *Hijra* groups in India can earn fees from performances at weddings and other ritual occasions. Work in these industries is not well-paid, and jobs are certainly not secure; economic pressure is chronic. The same is true for sex work, the economic base for many trans women and a few trans men. This provides an income, though rarely much more than a precarious living, not even tax-free if we count payoffs to police, landlords and gangs as a kind of tax. The clients often prefer youth, so sex workers, trans or otherwise, are likely to earn less as they grow older.

Since sex work is widely disrespected, the involvement of many transsexual women, *travestis* and *hijra* in the trade is a source of collective stigma for feminine trans groups, who are then liable to be portrayed as a source of pollution and disease. Hence the rhetoric of 'social cleansing', and occasional moral-panic campaigns by local government officials to drive the polluters out. Hostile cultural pressure is certainly not universal. *Hijra* for instance have a legitimate role in the ritual life of many local communities in South Asia, though there are also tensions around their presence.

Hostility can be ramped up by state and religious authorities. Organised hostility to trans groups is now a feature of the political landscape, more prominent than it was 20 years ago. Right-wing networks in the Catholic church, with support from the Vatican, have mounted campaigns in Europe and in Latin America against trans existence alongside denunciations of homosexuality, feminism and even the concept of 'gender' (Bracke & Paternotte, 2016; Garbagnoli & Prearo, 2017). In 2020 the right-wing Orbán government of Hungary used the COVID-19 crisis to push through a law repealing legal recognition of gender transition. Anti-homosexual legislation in Uganda and Nigeria impinge on trans groups too. I hate to think of the mental-health consequences of these populist manoeuvres; I know of no research on the question.

Making transitions work

In a discussion of transsexual women and feminism (Connell, 2012), I emphasised that gender transition is not a simple, all-or-nothing event. It is a process extending over time. It builds on contradictions in gendered embodiment that occur in some form in many people's lives, coming to a head in trans lives because of the intransigence, not the fluidity, of gender. Transition requires complex and extended work to make effective. The point applies to other moves towards 'gender diversity' such as producing a non-gendered or non-binary life. Queer theory speaks of the performativity of language, and it would be nice to speak a new gender into existence, but regrettably there is a lot of hard work to follow. This labour occurs in multiple arenas – embodiment, family relationships, workplaces, public spaces, and more.

As Josefina Fernández (2004) writes about *travestis* in Argentina, the family is where the story starts. Some families are the scene of sexual abuse or an angry father. But other parents provide care and support, or other members of the family provide support. In the autobiographical narratives in Ruth Morgan, Charl Marais and Joy Rosemary Wellbeloved's fascinating collection *Trans: Transgender Life Stories from South Africa* (2009), it is impossible to miss the importance of families. Here the families of relevance include the ancestors – and they are a resource worth thinking about in many other situations.

Work also occurs in the arena of the body. What is conventionally seen through the medical model of 'treatment' may better be understood as collective work. This is perhaps clearer in contexts of poverty, as illustrated by research with *travesti* sex workers in Brazil (Vartabedian, 2016). Many search for, and use, black-market hormones. Oil or silicone can be injected to change the profile of breasts and buttocks. There are workers in the informal economy who are experienced in doing this. But the injected oil may not be sterile, and industrial silicone is much cheaper than surgical quality silicone. Injected semi-fluids can migrate around the body and deform it; some trans women and *travestis* die from this, or from infections. I remember being asked, during a group discussion in Brazil, whether we used silicone in Australia. I said no, thinking of direct injection; but I forgot about silicone breast implants. Which sometimes rupture.

Staying alive and staying well through a gender transition is likely to involve negotiation with state agencies, as Viviane Namaste (2011) has emphasised, including the police, the health system, welfare agencies where they exist, and political and legal authorities. These negotiations are often collective rather than individual, and they are sometimes successful. In Iran, for instance, gender transition is legal and has religious approval. Transsexual women engage in intricate negotiations with state agencies and doctors to make the system work for them (Najmabadi, 2014). In Argentina, a coalition of trans groups, NGOs representing gay and lesbian groups, supportive feminists and politicians from left or centre-left parties, promoted an advanced Gender Identity Law, passed in 2012. This legalised gender transition and allowed transitioning women and men to gain the documentation they need (Argentina Ministry of Public Finances, 2012). Collective action can improve the collective situation.

Reflection

I will conclude with some thoughts on the kind of action that might be adequate to address the issues discussed above. Global-North discussions of transgender health mostly operate on a set of assumptions currently embodied in the World Professional Association for Transgender Health, formerly the Harry Benjamin International Gender Dysphoria Association – named for the very sympathetic endocrinologist who was a pioneer of transsexual medicine in the United States. Historically this model began with medical expertise and an established professional/client model of doctor/patient relations. Other professions now have a larger role, some services operate through clinics rather than private practice, and greater patient influence on the proceedings is admitted. But the health-professional expertise remains central, control is mainly in the hands of service providers, and the relationship with clients remains basically individualised. WPATH's key document is called 'Standards of Care', a set of practice guidelines that is regularly updated and is published in many languages.

There have been various criticisms of this approach, including its residual links to a pathological model of deviance. To me, the fundamental problem is that the professional/client framework of action is simply incapable of addressing the biggest problems about transgender health on a world scale. As indicated in the framework of gender analysis proposed at the start of this paper, these involve economic, power, and affective relations as well as identity questions: poverty, homelessness, housing, unemployment, police or paramilitary violence, conditions in the sex trade, anti-trans populism or religious bigotry. These problems are most acute in the postcolonial world, but they are also important in the global North. The main pressures on transgender health globally are of a kind that requires a collective, public-health and political response, not an individual treatment response.

Therefore I suggest that the critical resource for improving transgender and gender diverse health is not professionalism, however benign, but activism and organising in struggles for social justice. That is a tough proposition in conflict-ridden societies, but new stories of activism keep emerging (e.g. UN Women, 2020, on Ukraine). Trans groups, all taken together, are a small and marginalised part of the citizenry. These struggles undoubtedly require alliances with other social forces. Much trans debate has been preoccupied with what separates trans groups from each other and from other groups and movements. Inventing the concept of 'cisgender' – which misses the contradictory character of *all* social embodiment – did a lot of damage here. Perhaps we need to re-focus on the situations, experiences and interests that we share.

Acknowledgements

I am grateful to all participants in the group discussions mentioned in the text. This paper builds on my chapter in Ahonaa Roy, ed., *Gender, Sexuality, Decolonization* (Routledge, forthcoming), where a more detailed discussion of some points can be found.

Disclosure statement

No potential conflict of interest was reported by the author(s).

References

Alcaldía Mayor de Bogotá. (2014). Bogotá Humana abre el Centro de Atención a la Diversidad Sexual más grande de Latinoamérica. http://bogota.gov.co/article/bogot%C3%A1-humana-abre-el-centro-de-atenci%C3%B3n-la-diversidad-sexual-m%C3%A1s-grande-de-latinoam%C3%A9rica

Argentina, Ministry of Public Finances. (2012). IDENTIDAD DE GENERO Ley 26.743 Establécese el derecho a la identidad de género de las personas. English translation online at Transgender Europe website. https://tgeu.org/argentina-gender-identity-law/

Bracke, S., & Paternotte, D. (2016). Unpacking the sin of gender. *Religion and Gender*, *6*(2), 143–154. doi:10.18352/rg.10167

Carreras Sendra, N. (2009). Sexoservidores – homosexuales – 'vestidas' en la ciudad de Puebla. In R. F. Macip Ríos (Ed.), *Sujetos neoliberales en México* (pp. 17–49). Puebla: Benemerita Universidad Autonoma de Puebla.

Castillo, D. A., Gudelia, M., Gómez, R., & Rosas Solís, A. (2010). Violence and transvestite/transgender sex workers in Tijuana. In H. Dominguez-Ruvalcaba & I. Corona (Eds.), *Gender violence at the U.S.-Mexico border* (pp. 15–34). Tucson, Arizona: University of Arizona Press.

Collyer, F., Connell, R., Maia, J., & Morrell, R. (2019). *Knowledge and global power: Making new sciences in the South*. Melbourne: Monash University.

Connell, R. (2007). *Southern theory*. Sydney: Allen & Unwin; Cambridge: Polity Press.

Connell, R. (2012). Transsexual women and feminist thought: Toward new understanding and new politics. *Signs: Journal of Women in Culture and Society*, *37*(4), 857–881. doi:10.1086/664478

Connell, R. (2021). *Gender: In world perspective* (4th ed.). Cambridge: Polity Press.

DFensor. (2012). Limpieza social: respuesta falaz ante la crisis social. Special issue of *DFensor: Revista de derechos humanos*, D.F. México, April 2012, 10(4).

Fernández, J. (2004). *Cuerpos desobedientes: travestismo e identidad de género*. Buenos Aires: Edhasa.

Garbagnoli, S., & Prearo, M. (2017). *La croisade 'anti-genre': Du Vatican aux manifs pour tous*. Paris: Éditions Textuel.

Kidd, J. D., & Witten, T. M. (2007). Transgender and transsexual identities: The next Strange Fruit – hate crimes, violence and Genocide against the global trans-communities. *Journal of Hate Studies*, *6*, 31–63. doi:10.33972/jhs.47

Monro, S. (2005). *Gender politics*. London: Pluto.

Morgan, R., Marais, C., & Wellbeloved, J. R. (Eds.). (2009). *Trans: Transgender life stories from South Africa*. Auckland Park: Fanele.

Najmabadi, A. (2014). *Professing selves: Transsexuality and same-sex desire in contemporary Iran*. Durham: Duke University Press.

Namaste, V. (2011). *Sex change, social change: Reflections on identity, institutions, and imperialism* (2nd ed.). Toronto: Women's Press.

Namaste, V. (2015). The impact of HIV in Parisian trans communities, 1980–2000: The relevance of history for critical epistemologies on HIV/AIDS. In *Oversight: Critical reflections on feminist research and politics* (pp. 77–107). Toronto: Women's Press.

Reddy, G. (2006). *With respect to sex: Negotiating Hijra Identity in South India.* New Delhi: Yoda Press.

Reiter, B. (Ed.). (2018). *Constructing the pluriverse: The geopolitics of knowledge*. Durham: Duke University Press.

Ritterbusch, A. E. (2016). Mobilities at gunpoint: The geographies of (im)mobility of transgender sex workers in Colombia. *Annals of the American Association of Geographers, 106*(2), 422–433.

Serrano-Amaya, J. F. (2018). *Homophobic violence in armed conflict and political transition*. Cham: Palgrave Macmillan.

de Souza, E. M., & de Carrieri, A. P. (2015). When invisibility is impossible: Body, subjectivity, and labor among *travestis* and transsexuals. *Journal of Workplace Rights, April-June 2015*, 1–11. doi:10.1177/2158244015585406.

UN Women. (2020). Anastasiia Yeva Domani: How a transgender woman in Ukraine fought for her rights and discovered the activist within her. https://www.unwomen.org/en/news/stories/2020/2/feature-anastasiia-yeva-domani-transgender-woman-fights-for-her-rights

Vartabedian, J. (2016). Beauty that matters: Brazilian *Travesti* sex workers feeling beautiful. *Sociologus; Zeitschrift Fur Empirische Soziologie, Sozialpsychologische Und Ethnologische Forschung. A Journal for Empirical Sociology, Social Psychology, and Ethnic Research, 66*(1), 73–96.

World Health Organization. (2008). *Closing the gap in a generation: Health equity through action on the social determinants of health.* Final Report of the Commission on Social Determinants of Health. Geneva: World Health Organization.

Index